Alkaline Diet Cookbook:

Cleanse Your Body with 150 Alkaline Recipes and a 7-Day Meal Plan to Balance Your pH, Be More Energetic and Prevent Degenerative Diseases

(Complete Guide Book for Beginners)

Emma Moore

Table of Contents

INTRODUCTION

The biggest culprit in the acidification of our body fluids and tissues is simply the fact that we don't eat enough alkaline foods.
The Western diet relies heavily upon animal proteins in the form of meat and dairy products. Another dietary favourite –sugar- is also to blame, whether it comes from fructose, glucose, or sucrose.

Sugar, unfortunately, is the fuel source for many unhealthy invaders in the body, such as yeast and bacteria. These organisms, along with fungi, feed off of the sugars and proteins we ingest. As a result of the process, they excrete a variety of toxins, many of which are acidic. This lowers the body's pH balance, causing our internal systems to exist in an acid state instead of the alkaline state that is required for optimal health.

Food is not the only cause of acidification, however. An overabundance of stress can trigger the release of toxins in the body, too. Environmental pollution can also be blamed for a portion of the acidification of many people's bodies. By adjusting our diets to include more alkaline foods, we can help to realign the body's pH balance.

When we replace those acidic foods with alkaline ones, we allow the body to work in far more natural state of being. Many bacteria, fungi, and yeast cannot survive in an alkaline environment. The same can be said for many molds and viruses.

 When they can't get a foothold for survival, they can't go about damaging the body with their lifecycles. While the idea of completely overhauling one's diet is intimidating, it may very well be the best way to improve overall health. On the other hand, there is nothing wrong with slowly but steadily introducing more alkaline foods while removing the acidic ones. Some changes are far easier than one might even expect.

CHAPTER ONE
Alkaline Diet

The alkaline diet is a diet based on highly depurative foods of high nutritional density, with a high content of alkaline mineral salts, green foods rich in chlorophyll, legumes, some whole grains and quality omega oils (seeds and nuts).

This type of diet promotes the consumption of alkalizing foods (80% is recommended) and recommends that the remaining 20% be non-alkalizing but healthy because of their nutritional properties.

A food is classified as alkalizing or acidifying based on its biochemical effect on the body. In other words, it is not the pH of the food itself, but whether that food increases or decreases the pH of our interstitial fluids when consumed. It is important to understand this concept well because food can be acidic, but this does not imply that it is acidifying, but it can have an alkalizing effect when ingested, as in the case of lemon. The same happens with most fruits, because although many are alkaline, their sugar content is very high and therefore they acidify us when we consume them....

How to know if we are alkaline?

The pH is the measure that will help us to know our level of acidity or alkalinity. The scale of the pH goes from 0 to 14. Starting from the base that the 7 is neutral, everything that is below will be acid and everything that is above will be alkaline. The consumption of quality alkaline water, moderate physical exercise and adequate rest, among other things, are essential to maintain our pH balanced.

All of this, together, is what will help us to strengthen our state of health, our level of energy and our physical and mental line star. Yes, it is true that changing our way of feeding ourselves is the easiest way to begin to alkalize ourselves and that it will allow us to perceive improvements in our health, energy, and beauty more quickly. But we have to go beyond what we eat, the key is a more holistic approach to the concept.

PH balance benefits us on many levels: it strengthens your immune system, balances your weight, improves your mood, increases your energy level, it also has a positive effect on your libido, on sleep and rest, on the beauty of your skin, of your hair ... the benefits are global and begin to be noticed quickly. All of this can be achieved by progressively incorporating small changes in our diet and in our lives, which will help improve the quality of nutrition at the cellular level and detoxify the body.

The pH Scale

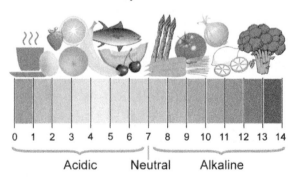

If we go to the most technical part of the issue about the effect of an alkaline diet, we should reflect on how the human body works and what role pH plays in health. The pH is a measure to check the acidity or alkalinity of a solution. When we measure the pH of our urine, we are obtaining information on the acid load (of toxins) that we are eliminating through it and, therefore, it will help us to understand how acidic our soil is.

What is acidity?

Each cell of your body, as a living organism, feeds and also generates metabolic waste (this process is called cellular respiration). These residues are expelled into the extracellular fluid and, obviously depending on the food received by the cell, the waste that it generates will be more or less toxic/acidic.

The importance of keeping the terrain clean and alkaline:

When the organism is acidified, that is if the metabolic waste of the cells accumulates, the blood loses its ability to retain and transport oxygen.

A cell under normal conditions gets the energy it needs from the oxygen of respiration, but the cells deprived of oxygen and in an acidic environment are in a limit situation that leads them, if they want to continue living, to look for any way of survival, in occasions, even mutating as a mechanism of self defense of the body.

By way of summary, we could conclude that a greater accumulation of waste, greater acidification, and a decrease in cellular oxygen is the ideal framework for diseases and pathologies to proliferate and thrive.

Albert Szent-Györgyi, Nobel Prize in physiology and medicine in 1937 for discovering vitamin C said: " The body is alkaline by design but its functions are acidifying ". This phrase comes to say, as explained above, that the body's metabolic processes generate acidity but the body needs an alkaline environment to function properly. But not only the body's own functions acidify, but there are many other factors that affect our pH: Negative emotions, lack of exercise, not drinking enough water or drinking it of poor quality, electromagnetic waves, medicines, chemicals, environmental pollution ... Unfortunately, we are surrounded by elements that acidify the body and that is why it is so important to compensate that acidity with a diet rich in alkalizing foods, exercising, with adequate rest, breathing with awareness to oxygenate well ... etc.

Benefits of the alkaline diet?

The alkaline diet is detoxifying: Promotes to take many fruits and vegetables which helps to purify your body.

Improve your habits: While other diets focus on food, the alkaline diet emphasizes your sleep and stress levels, improving your life in several ways.

Many people can feel better in cold weather.

The alkaline diet is perfect for weight loss: As you will see later the alkaline diet excludes sugar and refined flours.

What foods can / can not eat in the alkaline diet?

Foods allowed in the alkaline diet

Note: With allowed foods, we refer to alkaline foods, in foods that are not allowed, you will see acidic foods. Remember that the alkaline diet follows the 80/20 rule

Lemon Fruits (Except those that you will see in foods not allowed) Vegetables (Except those that you will see in foods not allowed) Seaweed Stevia Spices and condiments Apple cider vinegar Mineral waterBee pollen: And its derivatives Bean sprouts Almonds Chestnuts

Foods not allowed in the alkaline diet

Canned or dried fruits Blueberries Raisins Plums Cereals and their derivatives (especially those containing gluten) Corn Legumes OlivesPumpkin Butter Cheese Meats Eggs Fish Oils: Olive, sunflower, flax ... Aspartame Sugars of any kind Dried fruits (Except for those you saw in foods)

CHAPTER TWO
7-Day Alkaline Diet Meal Plan

PH levels show how much something is acidic or alkaline. On the pH scale, *0* is completely acidic, while *14* is completely alkaline, while *7* is neutral. Each individual body system has its own ideal pH level, while even small fluctuations in this balance can cause disastrous consequences.For this, you must take care of your diet.

Alkaline diet fights inflammation and overweight

Our blood is on the alkaline side, with a pH level between 7.35 and 7.45, while stomach acid needs to have a pH of 3.5 or less to break down food.To ensure the proper pH level of the blood, our urine changes its pH value. An alkaline diet is rich in alkaline foods to balance the pH levels in the body since modern diets are rich in acidic foods that promote inflammation and disease. Therefore, they prevent swelling, insomnia, poor memory, kidney stones, deficient energy levels, high blood pressure, headaches, diabetes, heart disease, muscle pain, and weak bones.

These diets are a popular trend these days, but despite this fact, they are a powerful tool against numerous diseases, including cancer.Many people report their positive personal experiences with these diets, but there are also many other people who can not understand how they work.

The medical community doubts the success of these diets because each body system has its own ideal pH levels. However, the facts show that an alkaline diet works and energizes the body and provides health and vitality. Alkaline diets are also compatible with weight loss, treatment of arthritis, inflammation, and cancer.

Namely, foods high in sugar and high in fat are acidic, they increase the acidity of the blood and the body extracts minerals from the bones and organs to restore the proper pH balance of 7.4. Acidity or high acidosis promotes inflammation and, therefore, causes diseases such as multiple sclerosis, joint pain, arrhythmia, immunodeficiency disorders, lethargy, and cancer. On the contrary, cancer cells can not fight in an alkaline environment. PH levels are also important for cell signaling, which is vital for your cells to perform their individual tasks.

These are the basic rules:

You should consume vegetables, most fruits, peas, legumes, beans, soy and tofu, some nuts and seeds, and many healthy fats such as olive oil, coconut oil, and flaxseed oil.

This is a list of the main alkaline foods:

- Artichokes
- Asparagus
- Broccoli
- Beetroot
- Date
- Figs
- Cauliflower
- Fennel

- Lemon
- Kale
- Spinach
- Watercress

On the other hand, you should avoid foods, sugar, dairy products, meat, eggs, alcohol, most cereals, caffeine, soybean, processed corn, safflower and sunflower oils, hydrogenated and margarine.

7-day alkaline diet Meal Plan

You must follow this plan and significantly increase your overall health. In addition, I also give you recipes for some simple, alkaline, but tasty meals.

As soon as you finish this week, try other delicious alkaline recipes from the chapter III of this book, or repeat this specific alkaline diet for another week and continue to improve your health. Remember to get enough sleep, exercise regularly and keep your body well hydrated.

Day 1

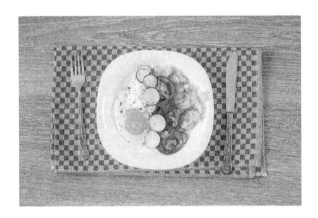

-Breakfast: *quinoa with chia and strawberry*

-Snack: *an orange*

-Lunch: *sweet and salty salad*

-Snack: *1/2 cup of toasted nuts and dried fruits*

-Dinner: *simple green salad with olive oil and apple cider vinegar, 3-4 oz. roasted chicken with roasted sweet potatoes and parsnips.*

Breakfast
Quinoa With Chia And Strawberry

INGREDIENTS:
- 1 cup cooked quinoa
- 5 tablespoons of chia seeds
- A ½ cup of strawberries in quarters + 4 sliced strawberries
- 2 chopped dates
- 2 tablespoons chopped almonds and grated coconut flakes without sugar
- 1 ½ cup of coconut milk

INSTRUCTIONS:
Cook the quinoa the night before, and in a blender, mix the dates and the coconut milk to prepare a puree.Pour into a jar and add the chia seeds. Stir well, cover with a lid and leave it in the fridge. In the morning, add the quinoa and chia seeds in a bowl and add the ingredients. Enjoy!

Lunch
Sweet And Salty Salad

INGREDIENTS:
- ½ cucumber, sliced
- 1 avocado, cubed
- 1 large head of butter lettuce, washed
- 1 pomegranate, without seeds or 1/3 cup of seeds
- ¼ cup pistachios without shell, chopped

Seasoning Ingredients:
- 1 clove of garlic, chopped
- A ¼ cup of apple cider vinegar
- A ½ cup of extra virgin olive oil

INSTRUCTIONS:
In a bowl, cut the lettuce and add the ingredients. In the end, add the dressing.

Dinner
Sweet Potatoes And Roasted Parsnips

INGREDIENTS:
- 1/2 kilo of sweet potatoes, cut into 1/2-inch chunks
- 1/2 kilo of parsnip / parsnip
- 2 tablespoons of olive oil
- Coarse salt and ground pepper
- 1 tablespoon of Dijon mustard
- Chopped parsley
- 2 tablespoons pure maple syrup

INSTRUCTIONS:
Peel and cut the parsnips, and preheat the oven to 230 ° C. Mix the parsnips in a baking tray with border, along with the sweet potatoes. Season with oil, salt, and pepper. Grill for half an hour, until they turn golden and tend.

In a smaller bowl, mix the mustard and maple syrup and pour the mixture over the vegetables. Sprinkle with parsley.

Day 2

-Breakfast: *vegan apple parfait*

-Snack: *1 pear*

-Lunch: *salted wraps of avocado and white bean stew*

-Snack: *1 handful of toasted pumpkin seeds*

-Dinner: *Simple cucumber salad with olive oil and apple cider vinegar. 100 grams of roast chicken with roasted brussels sprouts with red peppers*

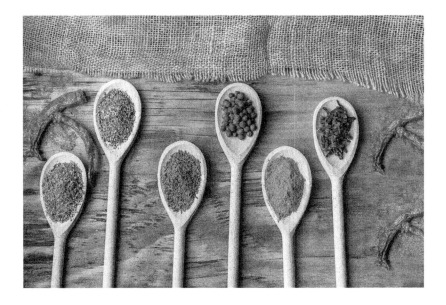

Breakfast
Vegan Apple Parfait

INGREDIENTS:
- 1 cup chopped apples
- 1/3 cup oat flakes, uncooked
- ½ cup of soaked raw cashews (soak 20 minutes-1 hour)
- ½ cup coconut milk without sugar
- ½ teaspoon vanilla extract
- 1 tablespoon of hemp seeds

INSTRUCTIONS:
Mix the coconut milk, cashews and vanilla together. In a small cup, place the ingredients in layers, first pour the cashew cream, then the apples and the oat flakes and hemp seeds on top.

Lunch
Salted Wraps Of Avocado And White Bean Stew

INGREDIENTS:

- ½ avocado
- 1 teaspoon chopped basil
- Small handful of spinach
- 1 tomato, sliced or chopped
- 1 butter lettuce or bunch of cauliflower leaves
- 1 teaspoon coriander, chopped
- ¼ red onion, cut in cubes
- Sea salt and pepper

INSTRUCTIONS:

Spread the avocado over the leaf, add the ingredients and fold it in half.

White bean stew

INGREDIENTS:

- 3 cups cannellini beans (white beans), rinsed and drained
- 1 3/4 cups chicken broth reduced in sodium
- 1 1/2 cups of chopped tomatoes
- 2 large cloves of garlic, chopped
- 1/4 cup plus 1/2 tablespoon extra virgin olive oil
- 10 cups of baby rocket loosely
- Baguette with 8 slices (3/4 inch thick)
- 1/4 teaspoon black pepper

INSTRUCTIONS:

Over moderately high heat, cook the garlic in 1/4 cup of oil in a large 3 1 / 2- to 4 1/2 quart pot for 1 to 2 minutes. Then, cut the tomatoes and add a little oil.

Add the pepper, the beans and the broth and put the mixture to boil. Lower the heat and let it simmer for 5 minutes. Add the greens and cook for a few more minutes, until it withers.

Dinner
Brussels Sprouts With Red Peppers

INGREDIENTS:
- 1½ pound of Brussels sprouts, small
- 2 plump garlic cloves (to taste), chopped
- 1 medium red pepper, cut into small cubes
- 1 tablespoon finely chopped lemon zest or grated salt
- 4 tablespoons of extra virgin olive oil
- 1 to 2 tablespoons of finely chopped mint (to taste)

INSTRUCTIONS:
- First, you have to cut the Brussels sprouts in the base, to get rid of the loose leaves. Then, cut them in halves and put them in a larger bowl.
- Add a tablespoon of olive oil and season with salt. Then preheat the oven to 200 ° C and line to tray with parchment paper. At medium heat, heat 2 tablespoons of olive oil in a large, heavy skillet.

- Add the sprout halves of Brussels, cut down, and sauté for 3 to 5 minutes until they get a nice brown color.

- Then, transfer them to a baking sheet, put them face down and repeat with the other shoots. Place the baking sheet in the oven and bake until soft, for another 10 minutes.

- At medium heat, heat the oil and add the red pepper, stir often and cook for 5 minutes. Add the garlic and cook for another minute. Add the roasted Brussels sprouts, stir again, and then add the mint, the lemon zest and the freshly ground pepper. Heat a little and season. Enjoy!

Day 3

-Breakfast: *Berry smoothie*

-Snack: *1 handle*

-Lunch: *Asian sesame dressing and noodles*

-Snack: *a handful of dried apricot*

-Dinner: *4 oz roasted salmon, ½ baked potato, curried beets and vegetables*

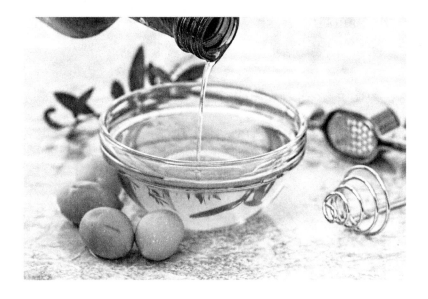

Breakfast
Berry Smoothie

INGREDIENTS:
- 1 cup of frozen mixed berries, strawberries
- 1 banana (peeled and frozen)
- 2 cups fresh spinach
- 2 cups of homemade almond milk
- 1 spoonful of chia
- 4 tablespoons of raw almond butter

INSTRUCTIONS:
In a blender, mix the almond milk and spinach, and then add the remaining ingredients, except for the chia. As soon as it is soft, add the chia and mix again at low speed. Leave it a few minutes for the chia seeds to expand

Lunch
Asian Sesame Dressing And Noodles

INGREDIENTS:

For the salad:
- 5-6 cups kale or spinach
- 1/2 cup of brown rice noodles
- 3 large carrots, cut into small, thin pieces
- 3 peppers, cut into small, thin pieces
- 400 grams chicken breast without skin without bone
- ½ cup of cashews or peanuts
- cup chopped cilantro leaves

- 4 green onions or green onions, only green parts, chopped

For the dressing:
- 2 large cloves of garlic, peeled
- ¼ cup of natural peanut butter
- ⅓ cup of soy sauce
- ¼ cup white distilled vinegar
- 2 tablespoons of honey
- 1 tablespoon ginger, chopped
- some squeezes of lemon juice
- ½ cup of coconut oil
- 2 tablespoons of water
- 2 tablespoons of sesame oil

INSTRUCTIONS:
- In a bowl of cold water, soak the noodles. Preheat the oven to 200 ° C. In a food processor, mix the ingredients of the dressing, pushing away the peanut butter.
- To marinate, add the chicken in a plastic bag and add ¼ to ½ cup of the dressing for approximately 15-30 minutes. In the food processor, add the peanut butter and press.
- Mix all the vegetables in a bowl. Bake the marinated chicken for 20 minutes, set aside for 10 minutes and then pour the vegetable mixture.
- Then, drain the noodles and cook them in a skillet over medium-high heat. Add a little oil, a little of the dressing, and stir while it is soft. Add a little water if necessary. At the end, garnish with crushed cilantro and peanuts.

Dinner
4 Oz Roasted Salmon, ½ Baked Potato, Curried Beets And Vegetables

INGREDIENTS:
- 1 bunch of beet / beet leaves
- 1/2 small onion, finely chopped
- 1/4 cup stems, finely chopped
- 1 tablespoon of coconut oil
- 3 garlic cloves
- 1/2 teaspoon of turmeric
- 1/2 teaspoon chili powder
- 1/2 serrano chili
- 1/4 semolina
- 1 cup of water
- 1/2 teaspoon ground cumin
- 1 tablespoon of lemon juice
- pinch of salt (or to taste)

INSTRUCTIONS:
- At medium heat, heat the oil in a pan and add the stems of beet, garlic, chili and onion. Cook them until the onions become transparent. Then, add the semolina and cook for 3 minutes.
- Add the cumin, chili powder and turmeric, and then the beets, salt and water. Cover the pan and cook for 5 minutes. Cook for 5 more with the pan uncovered, and stir frequently. At the end, sprinkle with lemon juice.

Day 4

-Breakfast: *Oatmeal and almond butter*
-Snack: *1 banana*
-Lunch: *Bowl with vegetables*
-Snack: *a handful of almonds*
-Dinner: *zucchini noodles and kale pesto*

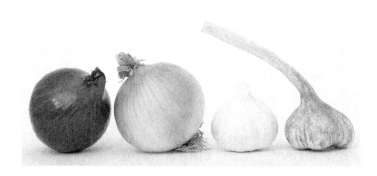

Breakfast
Oatmeal And Almond Butter

INGREDIENTS:
- 1 cup of grated green apple
- 1/3 cup of raw almond butter
- 2 cups of oatmeal
- 1 ½ cups of coconut milk
- a pinch of cinnamon

INSTRUCTIONS:
Mix the coconut milk, oats and almond butter in a bowl. Add the apple and transfer the mixture to a glass jar. Close with a lid and leave it in the fridge.In the morning, decorate with cinnamon and enjoy.

Lunch
Bowl With Vegetables

Ingredients for the dressing of avocado and cumin
- 1 avocado
- 1 tablespoon cumin powder
- pinch of cayenne pepper
- ¼ teaspoon sea salt
- 2 lemons, freshly squeezed
- 1 cup of filtered water
- 1 tablespoon of extra virgin olive oil
- Optional: ¼ teaspoon smoked paprika

Ingredients for Tahini lemon dressing:

- ¼ cup of tahini
- ½ lemon, freshly squeezed
- ½ cup of filtered water
- 1 clove of chopped garlic
- 1 tablespoon of extra virgin olive oil
- ¾ teaspoon sea salt
- Black pepper to taste

Ingredients for the salad:

- ½ zucchini, spiralized
- ½ cup of kelp noodles, soaked and drained
- 3 cups kale, chopped
- ½ cup of broccoli florets, chopped
- 1/3 cup of cherry tomatoes, cut in half
- 2 tablespoons of hemp seeds

INSTRUCTIONS:

- Steam the broccoli and kale and set aside. Then, mix the seaweed noodles and the zucchini noodles, and pour a generous serving of smoked avocado cumin dressing.
- Add some cherry tomatoes. Mix once more, and then steamed vegetables. Sprinkle with lemon tahini dressing, and then add tomatoes and noodles on top. Sprinkle with hemp seeds.

Dinner
Zucchini Noodles And Kale Pesto

INGREDIENTS:
- 1 zucchini noodles (spiral)
- 1/2 cup of nuts
- 2 freshly squeezed lemons
- 1 bunch of kale
- 2 cups fresh basil
- 1/4 cup extra virgin olive oil
- Sea salt and pepper
- Optional: sliced asparagus, spinach leaves and tomato

INSTRUCTIONS:
Soak the nuts the night before.The next morning, mix all the ingredients in a blender until you get a smooth mixture, and simply add the zucchini noodles.

Day 5

-**Breakfast**: energy shake

-**Snack**: an avocado

-**Lunch**: quinoa burrito bowl.

-**Snack**: a handful of dates.

-**Dinner**: wild rice mushrooms and almond risotto.

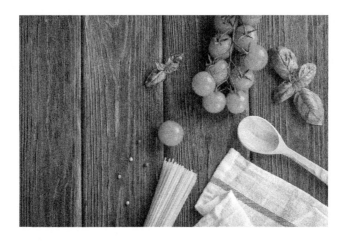

Breakfast
Energy Shake

INGREDIENTS:
- 2 cups fresh spinach
- 1 cup of frozen mixed berries
- 2 tablespoons of raw almond butter
- 2 cups of homemade almond milk
- 1 frozen banana
- 1 tablespoon of coconut oil
- ½ teaspoon of cinnamon

INSTRUCTIONS:
In a blender, mix the almond milk and spinach, and then add the other ingredients. Mix once more and enjoy it.

Lunch
Quinoa Burrito Bowl

INGREDIENTS:

- 1 cup of quinoa
- 4 sliced green onions
- 2 cans of black beans or adzuki.
- 4 cloves of garlic, chopped.
- 2 limes, fresh juice.
- 2 avocados, sliced.
- 1 spoonful of cumin.
- A small handful of coriander, chopped.

INSTRUCTIONS:

Cook the quinoa, and in a large skillet, heat the beans over low heat. Add the lime juice, cumin, garlic and onion, and cook for 10 to 15 minutes. Add fresh cilantro and avocado on top.

Dinner
Wild Rice Mushrooms And Almond Risotto

INGREDIENTS:

- 1.5 cups uncooked brown rice
- 2 cups of vegetable broth
- ½ cup sliced green onions
- 1 tablespoon of extra virgin olive oil
- ½ cup of raw walnut halves
- 1.5 cups chopped celery
- ½ of yellow onion; cut
- 4 medium white whole mushrooms; sliced
- 2 cloves of garlic, chopped
- Salt and pepper to taste

INSTRUCTIONS:

- In a medium skillet, sauté the mushrooms, onion, garlic and a cup of celery, stir and cook until the celery and onion are tender. Add the broth and brown rice, and boil.
- Lower the heat, simmer, cover the pan and cook for an hour. Stir for 30 minutes. Remove the rice from the heat when finished, remove the lid and add the green onions, and ½ cup of chopped celery.
- Next, set the oven to 180 ° C and line a baking sheet with parchment paper. Then, spread the nuts and toast for 8-10 minutes, turning them in half. When finished, cut the pecans and add them to the risotto.

Day 6

Breakfast: *breakfast pudding with chía.*

Snack: *½ cup of blueberries.*

Lunch: *miso soup with fermented tofu.*

Snack: *a handful of macadamia nuts.*

Dinner: *roasted root vegetables with 4 oz. Of salmon.*

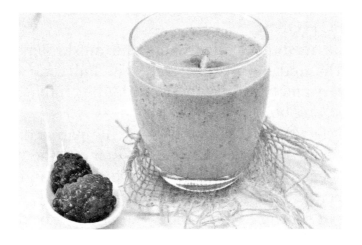

Breakfast
Breakfast Pudding With Chía

INGREDIENTS:
- 1 cup of coconut milk
- 4 tablespoons of chia seeds
- ½ teaspoon vanilla extract
- ¼ cup chopped walnuts (almonds, cashews or hazelnuts)
- ½ teaspoon of cinnamon
- 1 spoonful of grated coconut flakes without sugar

INSTRUCTIONS:
In a glass jar with lid, mix milk and chia seeds, add cinnamon, chopped nuts and vanilla.Then, cover it with a lid, shake it to mix well and leave it in the refrigerator.In the morning, shake again, add fresh fruits, nuts and pieces of coconut, and enjoy it.

Lunch
Miso Soup With Fermented Tofu.

Ingredients:
- 1/4 cup of firm fermented tofu, cubed
- 1/2 cup chopped green onion
- 4 cups of water
- 1/2 cup chopped Swiss chard or other tough green
- 1 sheet (1/4 cup) of nori, cut into large rectangles
- 3-4 tablespoons white miso paste

INSTRUCTIONS:
Simmer the water in a medium saucepan, and add the nori to cook for 7 minutes. In a smaller container, pour some hot water, add the miso and beat. Add the soup, stir and add the remaining ingredients. Cook for 5 minutes. Season and serve.

Dinner
Roasted Root Vegetables With 4 Oz. Of Salmon.

INGREDIENTS:

- 2 onions cut into 1-inch pieces
- 450 grams of parsnips, peeled, cut into 1-inch pieces
- 2 leeks (white and pale green parts only), cut into 1-inch thick rounds
- 2 tablespoons chopped fresh rosemary
- 1/2 kilo of red skin potatoes, unpeeled, cut into 1-inch pieces
- 1/2 kilo of peeled rutabagas, cut into 1-inch pieces
- 1/2 kilo of carrots, peeled, cut into 1-inch pieces
- 1/2 kilo of celery root (celery turnip), peeled, cut into 1-inch pieces
- 2 leeks (white and pale green parts only), cut into 1-inch thick rounds
- 1/2 cup olive oil
- 10 cloves of garlic, peeled
- Olive oil

INSTRUCTIONS:

- Place one grid in a lower third of the oven and another in the center. Preheat to 200 ° C. Cover 2 baking trays with olive oil. In a bowl, mix the ingredients, except garlic. Mix, season with salt and pepper, and divide the mixture between the trays. Grill for half an hour and stir occasionally.
- Then, simply invert the positions of the baking trays and add 5 cloves of garlic to each one. Grill for 45 minutes.

Day 7

-**Breakfast**: *quinoa porridge.*

-**Snack**: *some slices of melon.*

-**Lunch**: *Mexican quinoa salad.*

-**Snack**: *a handful of dried coconut slices.*

-**Dinner**: *pumpkin soup.*

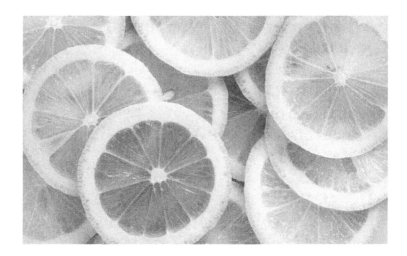

Breakfast
Quinoa Porridge

INGREDIENTS:
- ½ cup of rinsed quinoa
- 1 15 oz can of coconut milk
- 1 teaspoon of chia seeds
- 1 teaspoon of hemp seeds
- 1 teaspoon of cinnamon

INSTRUCTIONS:
Mix all the ingredients except for the hemp seeds in a small pot. Let them simmer for 10-15 minutes until the liquid is absorbed, and then sprinkle with hemp seeds.

Lunch
Mexican Quinoa Salad

INGREDIENTS:
- 2 cups cooked quinoa
- 400 grams of pinto beans, rinse and drain
- 400 grams of red beans, rinsed and drained
- 400 grams of shelled corn (optional)
- 1/4 cup fresh chopped cilantro
- 1 chopped red pepper
- 1 cup cooked brown rice
- 1 red onion, chopped

Dressing:
- 2 cloves of pureed garlic
- 1 tablespoon chili powder, or to taste
- 3/4 cup olive oil
- 1/3 cup of red wine vinegar
- 1/2 teaspoon ground black pepper
- 1/4 teaspoon of cayenne pepper, or to taste
- 1/2 teaspoon salt

INSTRUCTIONS:
In a glass bowl, mix the corn, pepper, cilantro, quinoa, pinto beans, red beans, red onion and brown rice.Beat the dressing and pour over this mixture.Mix and cover with a lid.Leave it in the fridge for 2 hours.

Dinner
Pumpkin Soup

INGREDIENTS:

- 3 cloves garlic, chopped
- 2 pumpkins (450 g pumpkin puree)
- 2 shallots, cut in cubes
- 1 cup light coconut milk
- 2 tablespoons of maple syrup or honey
- 2 cups of vegetable broth
- 1/4 teaspoon each: sea salt, nutmeg, black pepper, cinnamon

INSTRUCTIONS:

- First, preheat the oven to 176 ° C and line a baking sheet with parchment paper. Cut the top of 2 sugar pumpkins and cut them in half. Scrape all the seeds and tissue with a spoon.
- Brush the meat with oil and place it face down on the baking sheet. Bake for 45-50 minutes and remove from the oven. Let them cool for 10 minutes and peel off the skin.

- In a pan, add a tablespoon of olive oil, garlic and shallots, and cook for a few minutes. Add the rest of the ingredients, including the pumpkin, and simmer.
- Pour the soup in a blender and mix to make a puree. Then, return it to the pot, cook it for 5-10 more minutes and season it. Enjoy!

CHAPTER THREE
The Recipes

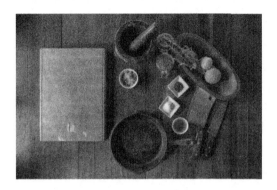

N ow that you know how to do an alkaline diet meal plan you can choose from a vaiety of recipes included in this chapter.

You will find four section: Breakfast recipes, Lunch Recipes, Dinner Recipes and Smoothie Recipes.
Enjoy!

BREAKFAST RECIPES

1. Strawberry Banana Smoothie

This amazing strawberry banana smoothie is simple and delicious, and you can take it to the next level with these flavor variations. Try them all! They're awesome.

INGREDIENTS:

- 2 cups frozen strawberries
- 1 fresh banana, peeled
- 1 cup milk (I prefer almond milk in this one)
- 1 cup Ice
- 1 tablespoon honey, if needed to sweeten

DIRECTIONS:

- Add all ingredients to a blender, and pulse until combined. Serve immediately.
- (If the smoothie is too thick, add more milk. If it is too thin, add more fruit and/or ice.)

2. Grain-Free Low Carb Cereal

Make this delicious low carb cereal from the 7-Day Raw Cleanse in 5 minutes.This recipe is raw, vegan, grain-free, and gluten-free, and full of protein.

INGREDIENTS:

- 2 tablespoons sliced raw almonds
- 2 tablespoons crushed raw walnuts

- 1 tablespoon raw sunflower seeds
- 1 tablespoon raw pumpkin seeds
- 1 tablespoon raw shelled hemp seeds
- 1 small green apple, cored and diced (See notes for Body Ecology)
- 1/4 teaspoon ground cinnamon, plus more to taste
- Pinch of Celtic sea salt
- Unsweetened almond milk, to serve (or any other milk)

INSTRUCTIONS

- In a bowl, combine the almonds, walnuts, sunflower seeds, pumpkin seeds, hemp seeds, apple, cinnamon, and salt. Pour the almond milk into the bowl, and add cinnamon to taste

3. Pineapple Orange Ginger Beet Smoothie

This amazing pineapple orange ginger beet smoothie from The Decadent Detox is so delicious it will make you excited to use beets in smoothies!

INGREDIENTS:

- 1 cup (240ml) filtered water, plus more if needed
- 2 medium oranges, peeled and segmented
- 1 medium raw red beet, peeled and finely chopped (grated for conventional blenders)
- 1/2 small avocado, peeled and pitted
- 1 1/2 teaspoons minced fresh ginger, plus more to taste

- 2 cups (320g) frozen pineapple
- 1/2 teaspoon probiotic powder (optional)
- Pinch of cayenne pepper (optional)

INSTRUCTIONS

- Throw all of the ingredients into your blender except the frozen pineapple, and blast on high for 30 to 60 seconds until well combined.Add the pineapple, and blast for another 30 seconds until smooth and creamy. Tweak ginger to taste.

4. Orange Creamsicle Smoothie

This orange creamsicle smoothie with oats and banana is an energizing and immune-boosting breakfast or snack that is vegan and gluten-free.

INGREDIENTS:

- 1 natural skimmed yogurt or vanilla flavor (can be replaced by vanilla ice cream balls)
- 150 ml of orange juice
- 1 teaspoon of sweetener
- 1 tablespoon of vanilla extract
- 2 cookie-type maria
- 1 teaspoon orange zest

INSTRUCTIONS

- T riturar cookies with orange juice with the help of a blender.
- Next, add the skimmed yogurt, the orange zest, the vanilla extract and the sweetener . You can replace the yogurt with vanilla ice cream and the result is also very rich.
- Beat all the ingredients until a uniform mixture forms and is slightly creamy.
- If you want to taste it very cold , add some ice cubes.
- Serve in glasses and decorate with mint leaves or sprinkle with a teaspoon of cocoa or orange zest .
- The ideal is to consume it instantly, so that it does not lose its freshness or diminish its properties. Otherwise, take to the refrigerator until serving time.
- This orange cream shake is not only tempting, but very nutritious from every point of view. Do not wait to prepare it at home! With very few ingredients and without major expenses, you will be serving an extremely natural and nutritious option to your family.

5. Strawberry Rose Almond Milk

This strawberry almond milk with rose water is super easy, absolutely delicious, and loaded with nutrients. This recipe is raw, vegan, and paleo friendly.

INGREDIENTS:

- 1 cup raw almonds, soaked for 12 hours
- 3 cups filtered water

- 1/4 cup chopped pitted dates (see notes for sugar-free option)
- 3 cups fresh strawberries
- 2 teaspoons pure rosewater, plus more to taste
- Pinch of Celtic sea salt

INSTRUCTIONS

- To soak the almonds, place the nuts in a glass or ceramic bowl or large glass jar, and cover with filtered water. Add 1 teaspoon Celtic sea salt and splash of fresh lemon juice or apple cider vinegar. Cover the container with a breathable kitchen towel, and allow to soak at room temperature for 12 hours.
- Drain, and discard the soaking liquid (do not use this to make the milk). Rinse the almonds several times to remove the anti-nutrients and enzyme inhibitors.
- Throw the rinsed almonds and clean filtered water into your blender, and blast on high for 30 to 60 seconds, until the nuts are completely pulverized.
- To strain, place a nut milk bag or knee-high piece of sheer nylon hosiery over the opening of a glass bowl, jar or jug. Pour the milk into the bag, twisting the bag closed, and gently squeezing it to pass the liquid through. Empty the almond pulp. (You can dehydrate this for use in smoothies, or to make crusts or body scrub.)
- Rinse your blender container, pour the strained milk back in, and add the strawberries, dates, rosewater, and salt. Blast on high for 30 to 60 seconds until smooth and creamy.
- Store the milk in a sealed container in the fridge. Activated almond milk (made with soaked almonds)

will keep for 2 to 3 days in a very cold fridge.

6. *Vegan Tofu Benedict*

This tofu benedict is vegan and gluten free, and only takes 15 minutes to make. This is a delicious, super easy vegan breakfast the whole family can enjoy.

INGREDIENTS

For the Tofu

- 1 14-ounce package extra firm tofu drained and pressed
- 2 tablespoons tamari
- 2 tablespoons apple cider vinegar
- 3 tablespoons nutritional yeast
- 1 teaspoon turmeric
- 1 teaspoon onion powder
- 1 teaspoon garlic powder
- ½ teaspoon sea salt
- ½ teaspoon black pepper

For the Hollandaise Sauce

- ½ cup raw cashews soaked in water for 2 hours, drained, and rinsed
- ¼ cup water
- 2 tablespoons nutritional yeast flakes
- 1½ tablespoons lemon juice
- 2 teaspoons Dijon mustard
- 1 teaspoon garlic powder
- ½ teaspoon ground turmeric

- ½ teaspoon sea salt

For the Benedicts

- 4 whole grain English muffins cut in half
- 1 large tomato sliced into 8 thin slices
- 4 cups baby spinach, baby kale, or arugula
- 8 slices tempeh bacon cooked

INSTRUCTIONS

To Make the Tofu

- If you're cooking the tofu in your oven, preheat it to 400°F and line a baking sheet with parchment paper.
- Cut the tofu in half, then cut each half into four slices. Place the slices in a shallow dish.
- Mix the tamari and apple cider vinegar together and pour it over the tofu. Make sure the pieces are totally submerged. Allow the tofu to marinate for 10 to 15 minutes.
- In a small bowl, whisk together the nutritional yeast, turmeric, onion powder, garlic powder, sea salt, and black pepper.
- Dip a tofu slice into the nutritional mixture and make sure it's fully coated. Place it on the baking sheet. Repeat with the rest of the tofu.
- Oven instructions: Bake the tofu for 20 minutes, flipping the slabs over after 10 minutes.
- Air fryer instructions: Bake the tofu on 400° for 10 minutes, flipping after 5 minutes. Depending on the size of your air fryer, you may need to cook the tofu in batches.

To Make the Hollandaise Sauce

- Mix all of the ingredients together in a food processor or high-speed blender until smooth and creamy. If it's too thick, add a little more water, a tablespoon at a time.
- Heat the sauce in a small sauce pan to warm it up. If it gets too thick, add a little more water, a tablespoon at a time.

To Make the Benedicts

- Toast the English muffins.
- Place two English muffin halves on a plate.
- Place about half a cup of greens on each half, then follow with a tomato slice and two slices of tempeh bacon.
- Place a tofu slice on each muffin half, and then drizzle on the hollandaise sauce. Serve hot.

7. *Vegan Lime Coconut Rice Pudding*

This easy vegan coconut rice pudding with lime and berries is gluten-free. Use cooked brown rice and your blender to throw this together in 15 minutes!

INGREDIENTS

- 1 3/4 cups (420ml) full-fat canned coconut milk (1 (13.5oz/400ml) can)
- 1 cup (70g) unsweetened shredded coconut
- 1/4 cup (60ml) pure maple syrup
- 1/4 teaspoon finely grated lime zest
- 1/4 cup (60ml) fresh lime juice

- 2 tablespoons minced ginger
- 2 teaspoons natural vanilla extract
- Pinch of Celtic sea salt
- 3 cups (450g) cooked brown rice (soft but not mushy)
- 3 tablespoons virgin coconut oil
- 1 cup (160g) fresh raspberries
- 1/4 cup (15g) coconut flakes

INSTRUCTIONS

- Pour 1 cup (240ml) of the coconut milk, the shredded coconut, maple syrup, lime zest, lime juice, ginger, vanilla, and salt into the blender jar of the KitchenAid® Pro Line® blender, secure the lid, and blast on high for 30 to 60 seconds, until smooth and creamy.
- Add 1 1/2 cups (225g) of the cooked rice, secure the lid, and process on variable speed 4 for 10 seconds, until creamy but rustic. (Be careful not to over process. You don't want the blend to be completely smooth or the porridge will be goopy.)
- In a saucepan over medium heat, melt the coconut oil, and pour in the blended rice mixture, and bring this mixture to a light simmer, about 1 minute. Reduce the heat to medium-low, and stir in the remaining 1 1/2 cups (225g) of cooked rice and the remaining 3/4 cup (180ml) of the coconut milk. Stir for about 2 minutes, until the mixture thickens slightly, but is still creamy and loose. (The mixture will thicken quickly while cooling for a minute, and if you cook for longer your porridge will get very dry.
- Divide the porridge evenly between four bowls, and top each bowl with 1 tablespoon of toasted coconut

flakes and 1/4 cup (40g) of fresh raspberries.
- Serve immediately.

8. Maple Walnut Baked Pears

These maple walnut baked pears are super easy to make with just 4 ingredients! This delicious dessert is vegan, gluten-free, and paleo friendly.

INGREDIENTS

- 1/4 cup crushed raw walnuts
- 2 large ripe pears
- 1/4 teaspoon ground cinnamon
- 4 tablespoons pure maple syrup or coconut nectar

INSTRUCTIONS

- Preheat the oven to 350°F/180°C.
- Line a baking sheet with a silicone liner or parchment paper.
- Cut the pears in half, then using a melon baller cut out and remove the center core with the seeds and place on the prepared baking sheet.
- Fill the pear cavities with the crushed walnuts, drizzle with maple syrup, and sprinkle with cinnamon.
- Bake in the oven for 20 to 30 minutes, until the pears are cooked through.
- Serve warm with cashew cream or ice cream.

9. Avocado Toast with Roasted Eggplant

This vegan avocado toast with roasted eggplant and hazelnut dukkah is a show-stopper gluten-free dish for breakfast, brunch, lunch, or a quick easy dinner.

INGREDIENTS:

- 1 whole wheat toast .
- hummus of eggplant .
- ½ avocado .
- ½ tablespoon of extra virgin olive oil .
- peppers.
- 1 boiled egg (optional).

INSTRUCTIONS

- Preheat your oven to 375°F/190°C.
- Line a baking tray with parchment paper or a non-stick sheet, and place the eggplant halves cut side up and the garlic cloves on the tray. Brush each eggplant piece with 1 tablespoon of olive oil and 1/8 teaspoon of salt.
- Roast the eggplant and garlic for about 30 minutes, until the eggplant is soft and golden.
- While the eggplant is cooking, make the dukkah. Throw the hazelnuts, cumin, coriander, thyme, salt, and cayenne into the small bowl of a food processor fitted with the s blade, and pulse a few times until the hazelnuts are roughly ground with a bit of texture. Transfer the mixture to a small bowl, and stir in the sesame seeds until well combined. Set aside.
- Once the eggplant is cooked, slice each half into bite-sized pieces, and squeeze the garlic out of the skins

and mash.

- Toast the bread, and assemble the toppings.
- Mash the avocado with 1 tablespoon of the lime juice, 2 tablespoons of the dukkah, and 1/4 teaspoon of the salt.
- To assemble the toasts, smear the roasted garlic on each slice, then the avocado mixture, top with spinach, eggplant slices, chiffonaded basil, a sprinkle of dukkah and salt, and a squeeze of lime juice.

10. CHAI-SPICED PEAR OATMEAL

This chai-spiced pear oatmeal is vegan and gluten-free, and is a delicious easy breakfast, dessert, or snack. Use a ripe pear for the sweetest flavor.

INGREDIENTS

- 1 chai spiced tea bag steeped in half a cup of hot water
- 1 tsp butter
- 1 bosc pear chopped
- 1/2 cup Quaker Old Fashioned Rolled Oats
- 1/2 cup low-fat milk
- 1/4 tsp cinnamon
- Pinch kosher salt
- 1 tsp vanilla extract
- 1 tablespoon almond butter

INSTRUCTIONS

- Prepare tea by steeping chia teabag in half a cup of hot water per your tea's instructions.
- Melt butter in a medium stock pot over medium heat.
- Add pear and sauté until brown, about five minutes.
- Add oats, tea, milk, cinnamon, and salt. Stir to combine and continue stirring until oats are thick and liquid is absorbed.
- Stir in vanilla.
- Portion oatmeal into bowl and top with almond butter.

11. Roasted Breakfast Potatoes

These roasted breakfast potatoes are super easy to make, and are vegan and gluten-free. The secret is the Massel vegetable powder and a blend of spices.

INGREDIENTS

- 2 pounds red potatoes quartered
- 1/2 small red onion chopped
- 1 red bell pepper chopped
- 2 tablespoons olive oil
- 1 teaspoon garlic powder
- 1 teaspoon kosher salt
- 1/2 teaspoon paprika
- Freshly ground black pepper to taste

INSTRUCTIONS

- Preheat oven to 425 degrees F.
- Place the potatoes, onion, and red pepper on a large baking sheet. Drizzle with olive oil and toss until

vegetables are well coated.

- In a small bowl, combine garlic powder, salt, and paprika. Sprinkle the seasonings over the vegetables and toss again until well coated. Season with freshly ground black pepper, to taste.
- Place the pan in the preheated oven and roast until potatoes are crispy, about 45 minutes.
- Remove from the oven and serve warm.

12.   *Mango Smoothie Bowl*

This mango smoothie bowl has a delicious tropical flavor that is just delicious.This recipe is gluten-free, vegan, allergy-free, and paleo-friendly, and makes an awesome breakfast or sweet treat.

INGREDIENTS

- 2 large mangoes (peeled, chopped & frozen)
- 1 cup coconut milk
- 1 cup almond milk
- 2 teaspoons honey
- 1 frozen banana

TOPPINGS:

- chia seeds
- fresh mango
- berries
- almond flakes

INSTRUCTIONS

- Place the frozen mango, frozen banana, both milks and the honey in your blender.
- Blend until smooth.
- Divide the mango smoothie between two bowls.
- Top with toppings of your choice.

13. *Blood Orange and Grapefruit Salad*

This blood orange salad with grapefruit and cinnamon is a simple but exquisite breakfast or brunch dish, and is raw, vegan, gluten-free, and paleo-friendly.

INGREDIENTS:

- The juice of ½ a blood orange
- 3 tablespoons of extra virgin olive oil
- 2 teaspoons of white wine vinegar
- 1 teaspoon of honey
- Salt and pepper
- ½ a red onion, peeled and finely sliced
- 2 blood oranges
- 1 pink grapefruit
- Feta or Whipped Ricotta
- A handful of salad leaves
- 10-12 black olives
- Pistachio nuts

INSTRUCTIONS

- If you are making the whipped ricotta you need to do this first and set aside.

- Next, make the dressing. Put the orange juice, olive oil, white wine vinegar and honey into a jar and give a really good shake to mix the ingredients together. Taste the dressing and season with salt and pepper as needed.
- Add the thinly sliced red onion to the dressing and allow them to 'cook' slightly in the dressing for about 10 minutes.
- Next peel and finely slice the blood oranges and grapefruit.
- Dress the salad leaves with a little of the salad dressing and arrange them on a plate. Put the finely sliced citrus fruit on top. Dot the whipped ricotta or crumble some feta on top of the fruit. Next, spoon a few of the onion slices and some more dressing on top. Finish with the olives and some pistachio nuts and serve immediately.

14. *Savory Green Smoothie*

This savory green smoothie with spinach and broth is vegan, gluten-free, and paleo-friendly, and is a a delicious cold soup that is loaded with nutrients.

INGREDIENTS:

- 1 cup water.
- 4 stalks of celery with leaves, chopped.
- 1 ripe avocado.
- 1 medium cucumber, with skin, chopped.
- Juice from 1 lemon.

- Handful of parsley.
- 1 clove garlic, optional.
- A pinch Himalayan salt.

INSTRUCTIONS

- Throw everything into your blender and blast on high for 30 to 60 seconds until smooth and creamy. Tweak cilantro, onion, lemon juice, salt, and pepper flakes to taste. Enjoy immediately.

15. *Vegan French Toast with Apples and Pecans*

This vegan French toast tastes just like conventional egg-based French toast but it dairy-free. I've used apples and pecans, but you can use any fruit!

INGREDIENTS

For The Flaxseed Eggs:

- 1 cup unsweetened almond milk
- 3 tbsp. ground flaxseeds
- 1 tsp. ground cinnamon
- 1 tsp. pure vanilla extract
- 1/2 tsp. ground nutmeg

For The French Toast:

- 4 slices thick wheat bread
- 1 tbsp. coconut oil

For The Cinnamon Apples:

- 1 tbsp. coconut oil
- 1 apple, sliced and chopped
- 1/2 tsp. cinnamon
- 2 tbsp. pecans, chopped

For Vegan Caramel Sauce:

- 3/4 cup coconut sugar
- 1 cup full fat coconut milk, at room temperature
- 1/4 tsp. sea salt

INSTRUCTIONS

- In a medium bowl, add almond milk, ground flaxseeds, cinnamon, vanilla, and nutmeg, and stir together. Let sit for 5 minutes.
- Heat coconut oil over medium-high heat in a large skillet.
- Dip a slice of bread into the flax egg mixture, letting it absorb the liquid, but not become overly soggy.
- Place bread on the skillet and cook until crispy and browned, about for 4-6 minutes.
- Flip and cook an additional for 4-6 minutes on the other side. Transfer toast to a plate.
- Repeat with the remaining bread.
- In the same skillet, add 1 tbsp. coconut oil. Add the sliced apples, pecans, and cinnamon, and stir to coat.
- Cook for 8-10 minutes, until softened.
- To make the caramel sauce, heat a sauce pan over medium-high heat.
- Add the coconut sugar, coconut milk, and sea salt, and stir to combine.

- Bring to a boil. Then, reduce to a simmer for 10 minutes, until caramel has thickened.
- Remove pan from heat, and allow to cool for 10 minutes. You can place in the refrigerator for 10 minutes to help cool and thicken.
- Top the French toast with the caramelized apples, chopped pecans, and caramel sauce.

16.   *Raw Vegan Plum Crumble*

This raw vegan plum crumble is super easy to throw together, totally delicious, and is gluten-free and paleo-friendly for a fantastic breakfast or dessert.

INGREDIENTS

- 3/4 cup pitted dates.
- 1/2 cup raw pecans.
- 1/2 cup raw walnuts.
- 2 tablespoons shelled hemp seeds.
- 1/2 teaspoon natural vanilla extract.
- Pinch of ground cinnamon, plus more for garnish.
- Pinch of Celtic sea salt.
- 5 fresh plums, pitted and sliced.
- 2 tablespoons pure maple syrup (or raw honey)
- Cashew cream, to serve

INSTRUCTIONS

- Combine the dates, pecans, walnuts, hemp seeds, vanilla, cinnamon, and salt in a food processor fitted with the s blade, and pulse until the mixture has the consistency of rustic bread crumbs. Transfer to a small bowl.

- In another bowl, toss the plums with the maple syrup until evenly coated.
- Divide the plums between four bowls. Spoon equal amounts of the crumble on top of the fruit. Serve with a dollop of cashew cream and a sprinkle of cinnamon. Serve immediately.

17.   *Lavender Almond Chia Pudding*

This lavender chia pudding is vegan and gluten-free, alkaline forming, and low in natural sugar.It's also a beautiful color and has a delightful flavor.

INGREDIENTS

- 1 cup raw almonds
- 3 cups filtered water
- 1/4 cup chopped pitted dates (or 5 drops alcohol-free liquid stevia)
- 1 teaspoon natural vanilla extract
- 3/4 teaspoon dried edible lavender
- Pinch of Celtic sea salt

Chia Pudding:

- lavender almond milk (recipe above)
- 1/2 cup + 1 tablespoon chia seeds
- 1/2 cup sliced raw almonds, to serve

INSTRUCTIONS

- To soak the almonds, place the nuts in a glass or ceramic bowl or large glass jar, and cover with filtered water. Add 1 teaspoon Celtic sea salt and splash of fresh lemon juice or apple cider vinegar, cover the container with a breathable kitchen towel, and allow to soak at room temperature for 12 hours. (For more information on soaking read here.)
- Drain, and discard the soaking liquid (do not use this to make the milk). Rinse the almonds several times to remove the anti-nutrients and enzyme inhibitors.
- To soak the dates, place them in a glass or ceramic bowl, and cover with filtered water for 30 minutes, until softened. Drain, and set aside.
- Throw the rinsed almonds, filtered water, dates, lavender, vanilla, and salt in your blender, and blast on high for 30 to 60 seconds, until the nuts are completely pulverized.
- To strain, place a nut milk bag or knee-high piece of sheer nylon hosiery over the opening of a glass bowl, jar or jug. Pour the milk into the bag, twisting the bag closed, and gently squeezing it to pass the liquid through. Empty the almond pulp and set aside. You can dehydrate this for use in smoothies or to make crusts. Or make this quick easy body scrub.
- To make the pudding, pour the milk in a large bowl, and whisk in the chia seeds for about 30 seconds to prevent them from clumping. Whisk again a couple of minutes later after the mixture settles to ensure the chia is evenly dispersed. Transfer the mixture to the fridge, and allow to thicken for 30 minutes.

- Stir in the almonds, and transfer to four bowls to serve. Top with additional sliced almonds, if desired.

18. Orange and Poppy Seed Muffin Smoothie

This orange and poppy seed smoothie tastes like a melted muffin. This recipe is vegan, gluten-free, and a seriously delicious breakfast!

INGREDIENTS

- 3/4 cup (180ml) unsweetened almond milk
- 1/8 teaspoon finely grated orange zest, plus more to taste
- 2 large oranges (or 3 small), peeled and seeded
- 1 medium-sized banana
- 1/2 cup (70g) raw unsalted cashews, soaked
- 1/4 cup (45g) rolled oats
- 2 tablespoons pure maple syrup
- 1 teaspoon natural vanilla extract
- 1/2 teaspoon probiotic powder (optional, see notes)
- Pinch of Celtic sea salt (optional, see notes)
- 1 teaspoon poppy seeds
- 1 cup (125g) ice cubes

INSTRUCTIONS

- Throw all of the ingredients into your KitchenAid® Pro Line® Series blender (except the poppy seeds and ice), and process on the smoothie setting, or on high for 40 to 60 seconds, until smooth and creamy. Add the poppy seeds and ice, and blast again on high for 10 to 20 seconds until chilled.

19.   *Tofu Scramble*

This tofu scramble with bell pepper and herbs really tastes like scrambled egg.This amazing breakfast or brunch dish is super easy, vegan, and gluten-free.

INGREDIENTS

- 8oz (~220g) Extra Firm Tofu
- 1 Tbsp Vegan Butter
- 2 Tbsp Nutritional Yeast
- 1/2 tsp Turmeric
- 1/2 tsp Paprika
- 1 tsp Dijon Mustard
- 1/2 tsp Garlic Powder
- 1/4 tsp Black Salt (Kala Namak)*
- 1/4 tsp Onion Powder
- 1/3 cup (80ml) Soy Milk

For Serving:

- Black Pepper
- Chopped Chives
- Fried Tomatoes
- Sliced Avocado

INSTRUCTIONS

- Mash the tofu with a fork but leave some nice big chunks.
- Add the nutritional yeast, turmeric, paprika, dijon mustard, garlic powder, black salt and onion powder to a bowl. Then add the soy milk and whisk it in so you have a nice sauce.
- Add the vegan butter to a frying pan and heat until hot. Add the tofu and fry it until lightly browned, being careful not to break it up too much when moving it around the pan.
- Add the sauce and fold it in. Fry it until you've achieved desired consistency, the tofu will absorb the sauce so you can have it as wet or as dry as you like.
- Top with some black pepper and chopped chives and serve with some fried tomatoes and sliced avocado.

20.   BERRY BEET SMOOTHIE

This berry beet smoothie is sweet, delicious, and looks gorgeous. If you think you can't enjoy beets in a smoothie, this blend will change your mind!

INGREDIENTS

- 1 cup plant milk of choice or water*
- 1 frozen banana.
- 1 small beet, washed, peeled, and cut into sixths**
- 1 cup fresh or frozen strawberries.
- 1 cup fresh or frozen blueberries.
- Optional add-in: 1 tablespoon hemp seeds.

INSTRUCTIONS

- Throw all of the ingredients into your KitchenAid Pro Line, Series blender, and process on the smoothie setting, or on high for 40 to 60 seconds, until smooth and creamy. Tweak ginger to taste.

21. *Vegan Gluten-Free Chocolate Pancakes*

These chocolate vegan gluten-free pancakes are incredible. They have a light fluffy texture and taste amazing even before you add the syrup!

INGREDIENTS

Pancakes

- 3/4 cup gluten-free oat flour*
- 3/4 cup gluten-free all-purpose flour
- 1/4 cup almond flour* (not almond meal, OR sub more gluten-free blend)
- 1/3 cup cocoa powder
- 2 tsp baking powder
- 1/2 tsp sea salt
- 1 medium ripe banana (the riper the better)
- 1 1/2 Tbsp melted coconut oil* (plus more for cooking)
- 1 tsp vanilla extract (optional)

- 1 1/2 Tbsp maple syrup
- 1 1/4 cup non-dairy milk
- 1/4 cup vegan dark or semi-sweet chocolate chips

FOR SERVING optional

- Vegan butter or Nut Butter
- Unsweetened coconut or Coconut Butter
- Sliced bananas
- Maple syrup

INSTRUCTIONS

- In a medium mixing bowl, sift together all the dry ingredients, which makes the pancakes light and fluffy.
- Make the chia paste by grinding the chia seeds in a spice grinder. Whisk the ground chia with the warm water and starch until well combined. Allow the mixture to sit for a few minutes and it should congeal into a gloopy sticky texture.
- In a separate bowl, mix all the wet ingredients together. Whisk in the chia paste until well combined.
- Add the wet ingredients to the dry ingredients, mix, and then stir in the chocolate chips. If you like your pancakes on the thinner side, add a little more water to the batter. It doesn't take much to thin the mix, so be careful. You don't want your pancakes to become a runny mess.
- Heat your skillet to medium heat and dollop on some coconut oil or ghee. Scoop 1/4 cup of batter at a time into the hot skillet. Once you see bubbles start to form, it's time to flip these babies over. The trick with pancakes is to keep the heat high enough to cook

them through, but not so high that it burns the outside while the inside is left raw. Once you find the right spot on your stove, take note.

- Let the pancakes sit for 5 minutes before serving. This helps them firm up in the middle.
- Serve with your favorite toppings.

NOTES

- *If you can't tolerate oats, you can try subbing a blend of gluten-free flour and almond flour, but I haven't tested it that way and can't guarantee the results.
- *If nut-free, sub the almond milk for rice or light coconut milk. And sub the almond flour for additional gluten-free flour blend.
- *If oil-free, try subbing the oil with applesauce or 1 Tbsp (15 g) nut butter.
- *Nutrition information is a rough estimate for 1 of 12 pancakes without toppings

22.   *Matcha Smoothie Bowl*

This matcha smoothie bowl is vegan and paleo-friendly, and loaded with healthy fats, chlorophyll, healthy fats, protein, and has a sweet delicious flavor.

INGREDIENTS

Smoothie

- 2 peeled, sliced and frozen ripe bananas (~120 g each)

- 1/4 cup chopped ripe pineapple (optional // frozen is best)
- 3/4 - 1 cup light coconut milk (canned or carton)*
- 2 tsp matcha green tea powder* (I like this brand)
- 1 heaping cup organic spinach or kale (I like to freeze mine to make the smoothie colder!)

Toppings Optional

- Fresh berries
- Coconut flake
- Banana slices
- Chia Seeds
- Slivered roasted almonds

INSTRUCTIONS

- Add frozen banana slices, pineapple (optional), lesser amount of coconut milk (3/4 cup or 180 ml as original recipe is written // adjust if altering batch size), matcha powder, and spinach to a blender and blend on high until creamy and smooth.
- Add only as much coconut milk as you need to help it blend. In my opinion, you want this smoothie somewhere between scoopable and drinkable.
- Taste and adjust flavor as needed, adding more banana (or a touch of maple syrup or stevia) for sweetness, matcha for more intense green tea flavor, or coconut milk for creaminess (though adding more matcha powder adds more caffeine, so use your best discretion). Pineapple will add a little tart/tang, so add more if desired.
- Divide between two serving bowls (amount as original recipe is written, adjust if altering batch size) and top

with desired toppings (optional). I went with fresh raspberries, chia seeds, and coconut flake. Bananas would make a delicious garnish as well.
- Best when fresh, though leftovers keep well sealed in the refrigerator up to 24 hours.

23. *Banana Coconut Chia Pudding*

This banana coconut chia pudding is vegan, gluten-free, and paleo-friendly, and is a delicious breakfast or dessert recipe or a sweet snack.

INGREDIENTS:

- 1 cup almond milk
- 2 tablespoons chia seeds
- 2 tablespoons rolled oats
- 1 tablespoon fresh lemon juice
- 1 tablespoon maple syrup
- 1 teaspoon vanilla
- 1 banana
- 1 tablespoon shredded coconut
- 1 tablespoon raisins
- dash of cinnamon

INSTRUCTIONS

- Throw the coconut milk, maple syrup, vanilla, cinnamon, and salt into your blender, and blast on high for 10 to 20 seconds until smooth. Transfer this mixture to a glass bowl or large jar and stir in the chia seeds until well combined.

- Chill in the fridge for at least 3 hours stirring occasionally to evenly distribute the chia seeds.
- Once chilled, stir the mixture again, and add in 1 mashed banana.
- Transfer the mixture to 4 serving bowls and top with chopped banana and shredded coconut.

24.   *Savory Granola*

This savory granola is vegan and gluten-free with an incredible blend of spices. Enjoy as a trail mix, cereal, or to top salads curries, soups, and stews.

INGREDIENTS

- 1 cup (100g) old-fashion rolled oats, gluten free
- 1/2 cup (60g) walnuts, chopped
- 1/2 cup (60g) cashews, chopped
- 1/2 cup (60g) pumpkin seeds
- 2 Tablespoons (30g) sesame seeds
- 1 Tablespoons fennel seeds
- 1/2 teaspoon ground chili pepper
- 1/4 teaspoon chili flakes
- 1 egg white
- 1/4 cup (60 ml) olive oil
- 1 Tablespoon agave syrup
- 1/2 teaspoon sea salt

INSTRUCTIONS

- Preheat the oven to 350°F (180°C), and line a large baking tray with parchment paper.

- In a large mixing bowl, mix together the rolled oats, walnuts, cashews, pumpkin, sesame, fennel seeds, chili pepper and flakes.
- Add in the egg white, olive oil, and agave syrup. Stir well.
- Pour the mixture onto the prepared baking tray and bake for about 20-30 minutes, stirring 2 or 3 times. Remove from the oven when the granola starts to be golden in color.
- Pour into a glass jar or an airtight container and store at room temperature for up to 3 weeks.

25. *Almond Milk Chia Pudding*

This chia pudding with almond milk is vegan, and gluten-free, and really delicious.Top with almonds and berries or banana for a great breakfast or snack.

INGREDIENTS

- 2 cups (480ml) unsweetened almond milk
- 1/3 cup (57g) firmly packed chopped pitted dates
- 1 teaspoon natural almond extract
- Pinch of Celtic sea salt
- 1/3 cup (53g) black chia seeds
- 1/3 cup (53g) sliced raw almonds, plus more for garnish

INSTRUCTIONS

- Throw the almond milk, dates, almond extract, and salt into your blender and blast on high for 30 to 60 seconds until the dates are completely pulverized.

- Transfer this mixture to a glass bowl or large jar and whisk in the chia seeds until well combined. Chill in the fridge for at least 3 hours stirring occasionally to evenly distribute the chia seeds.
- Once chilled, stir the mixture very well again to evenly distribute the chia seeds, and then stir in the chopped almonds. Transfer the mixture to 2 serving glasses or bowls and top with chopped almonds.

26.   *Vegan Gluten Free Waffles*

These vegan gluten free waffles with buckwheat and oats are incredible.They have fantastic flavor and texture, are easy to make, and are allergy free.

INGREDIENTS

Waffles

- 1 1/4 cup unsweetened almond milk
- 1 tsp white or apple cider vinegar
- 1/4 cup olive, avocado, or melted coconut oil
- 1/4 cup agave nectar or maple syrup (or honey if not vegan)
- 1/2 heaping cup gluten-free rolled oats
- 1 3/4 cups gluten-free flour blend
- 1 1/2 tsp baking powder
- 1 pinch sea salt

OPTIONAL ADD-INS:

- 1 tsp vanilla extract

- 1/2 tsp cinnamon
- 1 Tbsp flaxseed meal
- 1/4 cup dairy-free chocolate chips
- 1/4 cup chopped bananas or other fresh fruit

INSTRUCTIONS

- Oil and preheat your waffle iron.
- Add all of the ingredients except the baking powder in the order listed to the container of your blender. Cover and blend on high until smooth.
- Add the baking powder. Cover and blend on low for 5 seconds or just until incorporated. Let batter rest for 1 to 2 minutes.
- Pour the batter onto the hot waffle iron. Cook for 4 to 5 minutes or to desired crispness.
- Repeat, oiling the iron between each waffle.

27.   *Dehydrated Beet Hemp Granola*

This dehydrated beet hemp granola comes from The Full Helping.This beet hemp granola tastes delicious, and looks absolutely gorgeous. Utilizing beets for both sweetness and color yields spectacular results. As Gena points out in her original recipe post, this fantastic granola is loaded with nutrients.

INGREDIENTS

- 6 large pitted dates, soaked for 2 hours, then drained

- 1 large raw beet
- 1/2 cup filtered water
- 1 tablespoon melted virgin coconut oil
- 1 teaspoon ground cinnamon
- Pinch of Celtic sea salt
- 1 cup rolled oats, soaked for 30 minutes
- 1/2 cup raw sunflower seeds
- 1/2 cup shelled hemp seeds
- 1/3 cup dried goldenberries (or dried cranberries or raisins)

INSTRUCTIONS

- Blend the beet, dates, water, oil, cinnamon, and salt in a high-speed blender until smooth.
- In a large bowl, mix the oats, seeds, and goldenberries together. Pour the blended beet and date mixture over them, and stir until evenly coated.
- Line two dehydrator mesh screens with non-stick sheets or parchment paper, then spread the granola in an even layer on each.
- Dehydrate at 115 degrees for about 12 hours, then peel the layers off the sheets, turn over, and place directly on the mesh screens on the wet side. Dehydrate for another 12 hours, until dry and crispy. (If you don't have a dehydrator, bake at 375°F (190°C) for 10 to12 minutes, or until browning but not burning.
- Store in a sealed container, and enjoy with almond milk or as a healthy trail mix.

28. *Grain-Free Granola*

This raw, vegan, grain-free granola from Kitchen Stewardship is loaded with nutrients, super easy, and really delicious.

INGREDIENTS

- 1/2 cup unsweetened coconut flake
- 2 cups slivered raw almonds (slivered almonds do best here)
- 1 1/4 cup raw pecans
- 1 cup raw walnuts
- 3 Tbsp chia seeds
- 1 Tbsp flaxseed meal
- 1 1/2 tsp ground cinnamon (optional)
- 2 Tbsp coconut, cane, or muscavado sugar
- 1/4 tsp sea salt
- 3 Tbsp coconut or olive oil
- 1/3 scant cup maple syrup (or sub agave or honey if not vegan)
- 1/4 cup dried blueberries (optional // or other dried fruit)
- 1/4 cup roasted unsalted sunflower seeds (optional)

INSTRUCTIONS

- In a small bowl, mix together the coconut oil, maple syrup, and vanilla.
- Throw the almonds into a food processor fitted with the s blade, and pulse just a few times until rustically broken up. Transfer to a mixing bowl.
- Throw the walnuts or pecans into the food processor, and pulse a few times until rustically broken up.

Transfer to the bowl.

- Mix the almonds and walnuts together, and add in the coconut, seeds, and spices.
- Pour the liquid mixture over the top of the dry ingredients and stir until evenly incorporated. Add the dried fruit, and stir until combined.
- Spread the granola in a thin layer onto two dehydrator trays fitted with non-stick sheets or parchment paper.
- Dehydrate at 115 degrees fahrenheit for about 24 hours until dry.

29.   *Raw Raspberry Jam*

This raw raspberry jam thickened with chia seeds from The Blender Girl cookbook is really quick and easy and tastes just like conventional raspberry jam.

INGREDIENTS

- 130 g 1 cup raspberries, fresh (if using frozen, give time to defrost)
- 3 tbsp chia seeds
- 1 tsp vanilla paste
- 80 ml 1/3 cup water
- 1 tsp lemon juice
- 1 tbsp powdered sweetener or more if needed

INSTRUCTIONS

- Pour the coconut water into your blender and add the dates. Blast on high for 30 to 60 seconds, until the dates have broken up.

- Scrape down the sides of the container, then add the chia seeds and one-half of the raspberries. Pulse on low a few times, just to break up the berries.
- Add the remaining raspberries and pulse a few times on low to get a thick, chunky consistency. If the jam is too tart, stir in liquid sweetener to taste. Go easy, or the jam will get runny.
- Chill in the fridge for 30 minutes. The chia seeds will thicken the jam, and the flavors will develop. The jam keeps in the fridge for up to 5 days.

30. *Brazil Nut Chocolate Milkshake*

This raw vegan Brazil Nut chocolate milkshake is loaded with selenium and totally delicious.

INGREDIENTS
- 1/2 cup Brazil Nuts
- 1 cup Cold Water
- 1 Medjool Dates
- to taste Pink Himalayan Sea Salt
- to taste Ground Cinnamon
- 1 tsp Cacao Powder

DIRECTIONS
- Throw everything into your blender (including any boosters) and blast on high for 30 to 60 seconds until smooth and creamy. Tweak cinnamon to taste.

31. Vegan Breakfast Parfait

This vegan breakfast parfait with berries and cashew cream is super easy, delicious, loaded with nutrients, and makes an amazing edible centerpiece.

INGREDIENTS
Cashew Cream:
- 1/2 cup (120ml) filtered water, plus more to taste
- 1 cup raw unsalted cashews, soaked and drained
- 2 tablespoons pure maple syrup, plus more to taste
- teaspoon natural vanilla extract, plus more to taste
- Pinch of Celtic sea salt

Nut And Seed Mix:
- 1 cup raw almonds
- 1 cup raw walnuts
- 1/4 cup raw pumpkin seeds
- 1/4 cup raw sunflower seeds
- 1/4 cup shelled hemp seeds
- 1/4 cup unsweetened dried shredded coconut

Berries:
- 1 cup fresh blueberries
- 1 cup fresh raspberries

INSTRUCTION
- To make the cashew cream, drain the cashews, and discard the soaking water. Pour the fresh 1/2 cup filtered water into the blender, and add the soaked cashews with the maple syrup, vanilla, and salt. Blast on high for 30 to 60 seconds, until smooth and creamy. Tweak water, sweetener, and vanilla to taste. Transfer to a sealed container in the fridge, and chill for a few hours to thicken.

- To make the cashew cream, drain the cashews, and discard the soaking water. Pour the fresh 1/2 cup filtered water into the blender, and add the soaked cashews with the maple syrup, vanilla, and salt. Blast on high for 30 to 60 seconds, until smooth and creamy. Tweak water, sweetener, and vanilla to taste. Transfer to a sealed container in the fridge, and chill for a few hours to thicken.
- For the nut and seed mix, throw the almonds, walnuts, sunflower seeds, pumpkin seeds, hemp seeds, and coconut into your food processor, and pulse just a few times until the nuts are rustically chopped but still chunky.
- To assemble, take two short wide glasses, and place 1/2 cup blueberries into each glass. Next, spoon 1/4 cup of the nut and seed mix into each glass, half of the cashew cream into each glass, layer on 1/4 of the nut mixture into each glass, and then finish each parfait with raspberries.
- Serve immediately.

32. *Vegan Blueberry Crumble*

This vegan blueberry crumble is hard to stop eating. A great healthy snack for the whole family.

INGREDIENTS
- 300 grams blueberries (fresh or frozen)
- 1 tbs cornstarch
- 1 tbs brown sugar
- 1 ts vanilla extract
- 2 tbs lemon juice

For the crumble:
- 1 tbs flour

- 1 tbs brown sugar
- 1 tbs ground almonds
- 1 tbs rolled oats
- 1 tbs sliced almonds
- pinch of salt
- 1 tbs vegan margarine (or butter), refrigerated

For topping:
- vegan vanilla ice cream

INSTRUCTION

- Preheat oven to 350°F/180°C, and grease a rectangular baking dish with coconut oil.
- To prepare the fruit mix, throw the apple juice, berries, and salt in a medium saucepan, and simmer on low heat until reduced. Stir the arrowroot into the filtered water until well combined. Stir the arrowroot mixture into the berries, and simmer for about 5 minutes, until thickened.
- Pour the thickened fruit mixture into the greased baking dish.
- To prepare the topping, throw the oats, walnuts, almonds, coconut, sunflower seeds, pumpkin seeds, and flour into a food processor fitted with the s blade and pulse a few times just until the ingredients are slightly broken up and combined but still retain a rustic texture.
- In a medium-sized bowl, mix together the apple juice, maple syrup, and vanilla. Stir in the dry nut and seed mixture until well combined.
- Spoon this mixture over the fruit, and bake for about 30 minutes until slightly golden and bubbling.
- Serve warm or cold with cashew cream or ice cream.

33.   *Berry Protein Detox Smoothie*

INGREDIENTS
- ½ cup frozen blueberries
- ½ tbsp almond butter
- ½ cup unsweetend vanilla almond milk
- 1 scoop vanilla plant-based protein powder (we use Vega One Plant Power or Amazing Grass)*
- ½ teaspoon fresh lemon juice (ok, if not fresh)
- water to blend

INSTRUCTION
- Throw all the ingredients in the blender, and blast on high for 30 to 60 seconds until smooth and creamy.

34.   *Melon Ginger Green Smoothie*

This melon ginger smoothie with arugula from Super Healthy Kids is really delicious. A healthy nutrient-dense green smoothie the whole family can enjoy

INGREDIENTS
- 1 cup (240ml) freshly squeezed orange juice.
- 2 cups (300g) peeled and diced cantaloupe.
- 2 cups (300g) peeled and diced honeydew melon.
- 1 cup (14g) loosely packed arugula.
- 1 medium tangerine, peeled and segmented.

- 1/2 medium avocado peeled and pitted.
- 1 (1/2-inch) piece fresh ginger root, chopped.
- 1 tablespoon flax meal
- 1/8 teaspoon Celtic sea salt
- 1 cup (125g) ice cubes

Optional Boosters:
- 1 tablespoon Bulletproof Brain Octane Oil
- 1 tablespoon chia seeds
- 1/2 teaspoon probiotic powder

INSTRUCTIONS
- Throw all of the ingredients into your blender (including any boosters) and blast on high for 30 to 60 seconds until smooth and chilled.

35.   *Mixed Berry Smoothie with Superfoods*
This mixed berry smoothie with superfoods is delicious, and packed with vitamins, minerals, protein, and antioxidants for energy, immunity, and detox.

INGREDIENTS
- 2 cups (480ml) unsweetened hemp milk.
- 2 medium-sized bananas.
- 1 tablespoon goji berries.
- 1 tablespoon pure maple syrup.
- 2 teaspoons maqui powder.
- 1 teaspoon wheatgrass powder.
- 1 teaspoon shelled hemp seeds.
- 1 teaspoon chia seeds.

- 1 teaspoon flaxseed meal
- 1 teaspoon hemp oil
- 1 teaspoon natural vanilla extract
- Pinch of Celtic sea salt
- 1/2 teaspoon probiotic powder (optional, see notes)
- 2 cups 320g frozen mixed berrie

Instructions
- Throw all of your ingredients into your blender and blast on high for 30 to 60 seconds until smooth and creamy.

36.   *Chocolate Banana Maca Smoothie*
This Vegan chocolate banana maca smoothie with hemp milk, chia seeds, and flaxseeds is loaded with nutrients and tastes delicious,

INGREDIENTS
- 2/3 cup almond milk
- 1 banana
- 1 scoop vanilla protein powder
- 1 tablespoon Maca powder
- 1/2 tablespoon cacao powder
- 5 ice cubes

INSTRUCTIONS
- Throw all of the ingredients into your blender (including any boosters) and blast on high for 30 to 60 seconds until smooth and creamy.

- Consume immediately, as the maca flavor intensifies when left to sit.

37.   *Rosemary Watermelon Smoothie*

INGREDIENTS
- 2 cups (500 ml) of water
- ¾ cup (185 g) refined sugar
- rosemary leaves about 10 cm long, minced
- 2 cups of lemon juice
- 1 medium watermelon, seeded and cubed
- 8 cups ice cubes

How to do it
- Boil the water together with the sugar in a small saucepan over high heat. Add the rosemary, remove from heat and let stand for 1 hour.

- Place half of the lemon juice and half of the watermelon in the blender. Strain the rosemary syrup and pour into the blender. Cover and blend until smooth. Strain over a jug and blend the rest of the lemon and watermelon. Pour into the carafe and refrigerate until it cools. Stir before serving in glasses with ice.

38.   *Creamy Mint Kiwi Spinach Smoothie*

INGREDIENTS

- 1/4 banana, peeled and diced
- 1 kiwi, peeled and diced

- Juice of half a lime
- 120 ml full-cream milk
- 50 gr quark
- 4 mint leaves
- 50 gr spinach

INSTRUCTIONS
- Throw everything into your blender (including any boosters) and blast on high for 30 to 60 seconds until smooth and creamy.

39. Tastes-Like-Caramel Peach Mango Smoothie

INGREDIENTS
- 2 cups (480ml) unsweetened almond milk.
- 2 cups (86g) firmly packed baby spinach.
- 1/2 medium-sized sliced banana.
- 1 tablespoon pure maple syrup, plus more to taste.
- 1 teaspoon natural vanilla extract.
- Pinch of Celtic sea salt,
- 1 cup (160g) frozen mango.
- 1 cup (160g) frozen peaches.

Optional Boosters:
- 1 tablespoon flax oil
- 1 tablespoon chia seeds
- 2 teaspoons lucuma powder
- 1/2 teaspoon probiotic powder

INSTRUCTIONS

- Throw everything into your blender (including any boosters) and blast on high for 30 to 60 seconds until smooth and creamy. Tweak maple syrup to taste to get the caramel flavor.

40. *Vegan French Toast with Apples and Pecans*

This vegan French toast tastes just like conventional egg-based French toast but it dairy-free. I've used apples and pecans, but you can use any fruit!

INGREDIENTS

Apples:

- 2 tablespoons filtered water
- 2 tablespoons pure maple syrup
- 2 green apples, peeled, cored, and sliced
- 3/4 teaspoon ground cinnamon, plus more to taste
- Pinch of Celtic sea salt

French Toast:

- 3/4 cup (180ml) filtered water
- 1/4 cup (27g) raw pecans, plus more to serve
- 1 medium banana
- 2 tablespoons pure maple syrup, plus more to serve
- 1 teaspoon natural vanilla extract
- 1 teaspoon ground cinnamon
- 1/4 teaspoon Celtic sea salt
- 8 slices gluten-free sandwich bread
- 1/4 cup (60ml) melted coconut oil, plus more as needed

INSTRUCTIONS

- To make the apples, pour the water and maple syrup into a small saucepan. Over high heat, bring the mixture to a boil (this should take less than a minute) until it bubbles. Reduce the heat to medium, and stir in the apples, cinnamon, and salt. Cook the apples for about 10 minutes, stirring periodically until the liquid is absorbed and the apples have softened, but remain firm and in tact.

- To make the French toast, set your oven on the lowest heat or the "warm" setting.

- To make the batter, pour the water, pecans, banana, maple syrup, vanilla, cinnamon, and salt into your KitchenAid, Pro Line Series blender, and blast on high for about 30 seconds, until smooth and creamy.

- Pour the batter into a large shallow baking dish. In batches, place 2 slices of bread face down into the baking dish, and soak for 10 seconds until coated evenly. Turn over and soak the second side for 10 seconds until coated evenly.

- Into a small skillet (that fits two slices) or on a large griddle that holds all of the slices over medium heat, pour 1 tablespoon of coconut oil per two slices of soaked bread and fry for 4 to 6 minutes on each side until golden brown and crispy on the edges. You may need to add more coconut oil once you flip the bread in order for it to get crispy with your skillet and stove.

- If frying in batches, transfer the first batch to the oven to keep warm, and repeat the process, cooking the remaining slices of bread.

- Serve topped with cooked apples, pecans, and a drizzle of maple syrup. Pass extra maple syrup at the table.

41. Cauliflower Fried Rice with Turmeric, Ginger & Kale!

This cauliflower fried rice is one of my favourite meals to make at home and it takes around 5 minutes to create.

INGREDIENTS

- 1 large cauliflower
- 1/2 bunch of kale (any variety, but I love tuscan kale for this recipe)
- 1 tbsp coconut oil
- 1 zucchini (courgette)
- 1 inch fresh root ginger
- 1 inch fresh root turmeric
- 1 bunch of coriander
- 1/2 bunch parsley (any variety)
- 1 bunch mint
- 1 lime
- 4 spring onions
- 2 handfuls almonds
- 1 tbsp tamari soy sauce or Bragg Liquid Aminos

Optional:

- 1 green chilli
- Instead of fresh turmeric & ginger, use 1 tsp of each powdered

INSTRUCTIONS

- Start by making the cauliflower rice – this is really simple – just break the cauli up into small florets and chuck into your blender or food processor and pulse until it's like rice. If you don't have the blender, you can just grate it and get a very similar effect.
- Now is veggie prep time, so thinly slice your kale, quarter and then thinly slice the courgette (zucchini) and roughly chop all of your herbs (discard the mint and parsley stems, but keep the coriander stems)
- Next, prepare your ginger and turmeric – firstly by peeling them (for easy peeling, just scrape the back of a spoon over the ginger/turmeric – sweet!) and then grate them into a large pan with the coconut oil.
- As this starts to warm, stir the coriander, mint and parsley into the mix too including the coriander stems.
- After 30 seconds, stir in the cauliflower and then the kale
- After another 2-3 minutes, add the spring onions and the rest of the herbs, the tamari/Bragg and stir through – and then remove from the heat – the total cooking time for all of this so far should be under 5 minutes – you don't want anything going too soft!
- Now roughly chop the almonds and stir these through, season to taste and add lime juice as per your preference

42. *Immune Boosting Recipe: Asparagus & Ginger Broth*

Immune Boosting Carrot Ginger Soup! Looking to boost your immune system this cold season? Try this vegan and gluten-free creamy carrot soup. Serves 2, the perfect lunch- ready in just 10 minutes!

INGREDIENTS

- 3 cups organic, gluten free vegetable bouillon (I like the Marigold brand)
- 2 cups of filtered water
- 1 1/2 tbsp Bragg Liquid Aminos (or GF tamari)
- 1 inch of fresh root ginger – peeled and grated
- 2 garlic cloves – minced
- 1 fresh red chilli, chopped
- 8 stalks of asparagus – chopped
- 1 large handful kale – chopped
- 1 spring onion – chopped
- 1/2 cup fresh coriander chopped
- Glug of olive oil
- 1 dessert spoon of coconut oil
- Cracked black pepper
- Himalayan salt to taste

INSTRUCTIONS

- Heat the olive oil in a medium saucepan over medium heat. Add the onion and carrots and cook until softened, about 8-10 minutes, stirring often. Stir in the garlic and remove from heat.*

- Add the slightly cooled carrots, ginger, orange juice, turmeric, vegetable broth, salt and freshly ground pepper to the NutriBullet Balance. Blend for 45 seconds until creamy and smooth.
- Serve! I garnished this with an extra drizzle of good olive-oil and freshly ground pepper.

43. Roasted Turmeric Cauliflower Kale Salad

A sweet and savory kale salad with roasted turmeric cauliflower and chickpeas.

INGREDIENTS

- 1/2 head cauliflower (washed, rinsed and dried)
- 5 stalks of curly kale or tuscan kale (washed and rinsed)
- 1 capsicum/bell pepper
- 1 stalk celery
- 1/2 avocado
- 2 tomatoes
- 1 tablespoon turmeric or 2cm fresh, grated
- 1/4 teaspoon cayenne pepper
- 1/4 teaspoon paprika
- 1/2 lemon
- 1/4 teaspoon Bragg Liquid Aminos or organic tamari
- Himalayan salt & black pepper
- Pumpkin seeds
- Coconut oil
- Olive oil

INSTRUCTIONS

- Preheat the oven to 355F (180C).
- Rip or chop the cauliflower head into floret an in a mixing bowl combine with the turmeric, cayenne pepper, paprika, salt and pepper and 2 tbsp of coconut oil and mix thoroughly.
- Line a baking tray with baking paper and spread the cauliflower and any of the seasoning out onto the tray and put into the preheated oven in the middle shelf for 20 minutes – be sure to check regularly to make sure the cauliflower isn't burning. If it is, move to the bottom shelf.
- Now, chop the kale from the stems and roughly tear or chop into pieces and place in a large bowl. Mix in the lemon juice and massage with your hands for a minute. Then add the Bragg's or tamari and place on your serving plates.
- Thinly slice the bell pepper/capsicum, celery, chop the avocado into chunks and roughly chop the tomato. Place these on top of the kale bed. Sprinkle with pumpkin seeds and drizzle a little olive oil over this.
- Once the cauliflower is done, remove from the oven and place on top of each salad and serve immediately.

44. *Summer Salad with Mint & Lemon Dressing*

This mint salad dressing recipe is refreshing, delicious and easy to make! You'll need fresh mint, lemon juice, olive oil,

Dijon mustard, and honey or maple syrup. Recipe yields a little over 1 cup

INGREDIENTS:

For the Mint and Lemon Seasoning

- ¼ cup olive oil
- ¼ cup of lemon juice
- ½ cup of disinfected mint leaves
- 1 teaspoon salt
- ½ teaspoon ground black pepper
- ½ cup of SPLENDA No Calorie Sweetener Granulated

For the salad

- 2 medium-sized washed zucchini
- 3 branches of disinfected celery
- ½ avocado (medium)
- 120 g of natural goat cheese
- 6 cups of organic lettuce

INSTRUCTIONS

- Start by preparing the asparagus, by blanching it (place it into boiling water for 1 minute and then drain and rinse under cold water asap) and then slicing along the length to create long strips.
- Next very gently fry the zucchini in a griddle pan (or regular pan if you don't have a griddle) until it's just starting to brown.

- Now begin assembling the salad by combining the asparagus, zucchini, avocado, cilantro, parsley, radish and peas in a large bowl.
- Make the dressing by blending all ingredients in a blender or food processor.
- Dress and season to taste and you're away!

NOTE: the dressing will keep for up to a week in an airtight container in the fridge.

45. *Quinoa Stuffed Spaghetti Squash*

This quinoa stuffed squash is such a wonderful, It's loaded with nutrients and plenty of plant-based protein.

INGREDIENTS

- 1 big or two smaller spaghetti squashes
- 2 tbsp. coconut oil
- 1 cup steamed green peas
- 1 medium shallot
- 1 orange or red bell pepper
- 2 spring onions, white part, sliced
- 1/4 cup chopped walnuts
- 1 and 1/2 cup cooked quinoa
- 2 tsp. dried thyme
- 1 tsp. garlic powder
- Pink salt and black pepper to taste

INSTRUCTIONS

- Preheat the oven to 400°F

- Wash the squash and slice them in half. Remove seeds and bake until tender, about 40 minutes.
- While the squash is roasting heat 1 tbsp. oil in a skillet and cook the finely chopped shallot and bell pepper until soft. Add spices, green peas, cooked quinoa and walnuts until warmed through. Flavour with pink salt and pepper.
- Divide between the squash and place back in the oven for 5 – 8 minutes. Remove from the oven and serve with fresh greens on top, I used broccoli and a big green salad.

- Spaghetti squash has a light texture which makes it easy and fun to eat, you can scratch the flesh with a fork and it resembles spaghetti.

46. *Crunchy Kale Salad with Tahini Dressing*

An easy-to-make, nutritious kale salad packed with roasted veggies, crispy chickpeas, and fluffy red quinoa. Tossed in a garlicky tahini-based dressing with lemon and basil flavors. GF, DF, and vegan

INGREDIENTS

- 4 big handfuls of kale, stalks removed and roughly sliced
- 8 brussels sprouts, shaved thin
- 2 radishes, thinly sliced
- 1 carrot, shredded or thinly sliced

- 1/2 cup of canellini beans (or any other beans you like!)
- 2 tablespoons of almonds, roughly chopped
- 1 tablespoon of cashews
- 1 tablespoon of pumpkin seeds
- 1 cup basil, chopped

For the Tahini Dressing

- Half a large avocado
- 1 tbsp tahini
- 1 garlic clove
- 1 tbsp olive or flax oil
- 2 tbsp fresh lemon juice
- Cracked black pepper
- Pinch of Himalayan salt

INSTRUCTIONS

For the Kale & Quinoa Salad

- Preheat the oven to 425 degrees.
- Toss the veggies and chickpeas with the salt, pepper, and avocado oil. Place on a baking sheet that has been greased or lined with parchment paper.

- Bake all of the veggies except for the cherry tomatoes for 20 minutes and the chickpeas for 40 minutes, flipping or tossing half way through (flip the veggies at 10 minutes and toss the chickpeas at 20 minutes).
- While the veggies are baking, cook the quinoa per package instructions (~20 minutes).

- After the quinoa is done cooking, massage the kale in the extra virgin olive oil (pour oil onto kale and rub the leaves together with your hands for 1-2 minutes). Toss the kale, quinoa, and cherry tomato halves together. You can make the dressing after this is done!
- When the veggies and chickpeas are both done cooking, toss with the kale mixture. Enjoy!

For the Lemon Tahini Dressing

- Blend all dressing ingredients in a small food processor or good blender (I use a Vitamix A2300) on a low speed setting for about 5 minutes.
- Toss over the salad. This dressing recipe makes about 2/3 cup. I toss 1/2 of it over the salad and save the other 1/2 in the fridge for the week.

47. *The Alkaline Immune Boosting Vegetables Soup*

INGREDIENTS

Cooked Ingredients:

- 1 brown onion, sliced roughly
- 2 cloves of garlic, chopped roughly
- 2 carrots, sliced
- 1/4 head of cauliflower
- 1/4 head of broccoli
- 1/4 head of cabbage (any green variety)
- 200ml vegetable stock

- 1 can of organic chopped tomatoes (or 8 fresh tomatoes)
- Himalayan Pink Salt & Black pepper to taste
- 1/2 inch of ginger root (or 1tsp dried)
- 1/2 inch of turmeric root (or 1tsp dried)
- Coconut oil

Raw Ingredients:

- 1/2 cucumber
- 3 tomatoes
- 1 handful spinach
- 1/2 bunch of basil
- 1/4 bunch of coriander
- 1/2 tin of chickpeas (garbanzos)

INSTRUCTIONS

- Start by gently frying the onions and garlic in a little coconut oil. After 3 minutes, throw in the carrots, cauliflower, broccoli, cabbage and allow to cook for another 3 minutes
- Now add the stock and tomatoes/can of tomatoes – allow to simmer for 20-25 minutes until the vegetables are softened a little.
- In the meantime, roughly chop the raw foods and put into a blender and blend until smooth
- When the soup has simmered for 20 minutes transfer it in batches (as much as your blender will hold) and blend it all together until smooth with the raw blended mixture too.

- It may take a couple of batches into the blender, but you want to end up with a smooth soup. Serve with a sprig of coriander or basil and enjoy warm!

48.   *Instant Alkaline Sushi Roll Ups*

INGREDIENTS

For the Dip/Hummous

- 100g of chickpeas/garbanzos from a can, drained or prepared from dried
- A handful of almonds
- 1 tbsp tahini
- 1 pinch of cumin
- A glug of olive oil
- 1 clove of garlic
- Juice of 1/2 lemon
- Pinch of Himalayan salt

For the Roll-Ups

- 2 medium zucchini/courgette (each will give you 5-6 rolls)
- 1 carrot sliced into matchsticks
- 1 cucumber sliced into matchsticks
- 1 avocado, peeled and sliced

- 1 small bunch coriander/cilantro
- 1 capsicum sliced into matchsticks

INSTRUCTIONS

- Chop the ends off of your courgette/zucchini and use a vegetable peeler to very carefully peel your zucchini into long, thin strips – please be careful of your fingers, I sliced the end off mine not so long ago! Then lay each zucchini strip out and spread a nice thick layer of the almond hummus onto the strip – enough for the veggies to stick to
- Add a few matchsticks of veggies, avocado, and a couple of pieces of coriander
- Sprinkle on the sesame seeds, roll up and ENJOY!

49.   *Wheat Free Quinoa & Hummus Wraps*

This hummus wrap is a great option for lunch or dinner — packed with protein thanks to quinoa and hummus, it will keep you full for hours.

INGREDIENTS

- 4 large Collard Leaves (depending on gaps you may need a couple more)
- 1/2 cup Sprouts (any you like)
- 1/2 cup Purple Cabbage, shredded or carrots
- 1/2 cup Beetroot, either cooked and mashed or raw sliced very finely

- 1 cup Quinoa
- 1 cup Hummus
- 1 cup Avocado

INSTRUCTIONS

- First, get the quinoa cooking - put the cup of quinoa into a pan with 2 cups of cold water, bring to the boil and then simmer on a really low heat until the water is evaporated and the quinoa is fluffy
- Next get the wraps going by prepping out the collard leaves, cut from the plant, washed and laid out like a regular wrap
- Next spread the hummous equally over each leaf - the hummous acts like a glue for the ingredients!
- Slice and lay out the avocado in a line from top to bottom down the middle of the leaf
- Add the quinoa equally between the leaves and then fill with the remaining ingredients
- Next wrap by folding at the bottom (to stop everything falling out) and then rolling into a regular wrap shape!

50.   Little Gem Lettuce Salad

INGREDIENTS

For the walnut vinaigrette

- 2 tablespoons fresh lemon juice (from 1/2 large lemon)
- 2 tablespoons Champagne vinegar
- 1 teaspoon whole-grain mustard

- 1/2 teaspoon kosher salt
- 5 grinds black pepper
- 1/4 cup grapeseed oil
- 1/4 cup walnut oil, plus more for drizzling, if desired

For the salad

- 2 large or 4 small heads Little Gem lettuce* (about 10 oz), cored, leaves left whole or torn in half, if large
- 1/2 cup loosely packed flat-leaf parsley leaves
- 1/4 cup roughly chopped dill
- 3 large radishes, very thinly sliced
- 2 tablespoons minced shallot
- 8 chives, cut into 1-inch (2.5-cm) pieces
- 1/2 cup walnuts, toasted and chopped
- 1/4 cup walnut vinaigrette, plus more, to taste
- Kosher salt and freshly ground black pepper
- 1 ounce ricotta salata cheese

INSTRUCTIONS

- Fill the lettuce leaves with the chopped salad ingredients and drizzle with the olive oil, a squeeze of fresh lemon and serve!
- That's all there is to it, it's as simple as that.
- If you want to increase the omega 3 content, you could swap the olive oil for flax oil, or make a mix of 50/50 of each. This tastes delicious too.

51. Turmeric & Lentil Anti-Inflammatory Soup

A warm bowl of comforting lentil soup, packed with whole ingredients (red lentils, root veggies, greens) and a lot of turmeric for its anti-inflammatory properties.

INGREDIENTS:

Soup:

- 200g Pumpkin, roughly chopped
- 4 Carrots, roughly chopped
- 1 Sweet Red Potato, roughly chopped
- 4 Tomatoes, roughly chopped
- 3 Cloves Garlic
- 1tsp Mustard Seeds
- 1 Red Onion
- 300ml Vegetable Stock
- 200ml Coconut Cream
- 1 Handful of Fresh Coriander (Cilantro), roughly chopped
- 1 Inch Fresh Turmeric Root
- 1 Inch Fresh Ginger Root
- 1/2 Red Pepper (Capsicum/Bell Pepper)
- 1 Cup of Lentils
- Coconut Oil

Optional Topping:

- 1/2 Cup Cashews
- 2 Tbsp Pumpkin Seeds
- 1 Clove Garlic, minced
- Optional: thinly sliced red chilli

INSTRUCTIONS

- Start by chopping the red onion, garlic, ginger (peeled) and turmeric (peeled) roughly.
- Gently heat a little coconut oil in a pan and very gently get the onion started, and once it's cooking a little, add the turmeric, ginger, mustard seeds and garlic – being careful not to burn the garlic.
- Now add the root veggies (carrot, pumpkin, sweet potato), the red pepper and the tomatoes and stir it all around to coat the veggies in the oil and flavours (you should be able to smell that delicious turmeric now)
- Add the stock and then add the lentils. If you're using dried lentils, you will need to add an extra 50ml of stock to allow for an additional 10 mins cooking time, but if you're using tinned lentils (please buy organic), add them now and move onto the next step.
- Turn the heat down to simmer and let all of the veggies soften and the lentils cook.
- Once everything has softened, add the coconut cream and chopped cilantro (coriander) and then transfer to a blender and blend until smooth
- This will stay nice and warm for about an hour in the blender jug, but if you want, you can return to the pan to keep warm
- To make the optional topping (which I've found really nice and a delicious extra texture to the soup), simply roughly smash up the cashews on a chopping board under a knife, and cook with the pumpkin seeds in a little coconut oil with the minced garlic until it's warmed through and a little browned.

- Serve the soup in bowls with a sprig of cilantro, a drizzle of coconut cream and the cashew topping (with optional chilli) and LOVE it

52. *Alkaline Springtime Soup*

INGREDIENTS:

- 1 shallot or small brown onion
- 1/2 cucumber
- 1 tablespoon of olive, flax or Udo's Choice
- 250ml vegetable stock (yeast free)
- 2 sprigs of mint
- 1lb or 450g of frozen peas
- 1/2 avocado
- Salt & pepper to taste

DIRECTIONS

- FOR QUINOA: Cook 2 cups of quinoa in a 'rice' cooker, or cook quinoa by combining 4 cups of water or vegetable broth with 2 cups of quinoa in a pot over high heat. When the liquid comes to a boil, cover the pot and turn heat down to the lowest setting for 15-20 minutes (until liquid is gone).
- FOR SOUP: Heat the vegetable broth in a pot over medium heat, add quinoa, garbanzo beans, and chipotle spice and heat through for 10 minutes. Add zucchini and squash and cook for 5 more minutes.

53. Rocket, Watercress & Mint Salad

INGREDIENTS

- 100g rocket (also known as arugula)
- 100g watercress
- 100g chickpeas
- 1/2 bunch of fresh mint
- 2tbsp of olive oil
- 2tbsp fresh lemon juice
- Himalayan salt and ground pepper

INSTRUCTIONS

- Wash the leaves and dry them. Arrange them in a bowl and toss through the chickpeas. Sprinkle the mint on top and then add the dressing, salt and pepper and enjoy!

54. Quinoa Salad

The quinoa salad is a very nutritious, healthy and light dish.It is a very easy and simple recipe.You can add your favorite ingredients.

INGREDIENTS

- 1/2 cup of uncooked quinoa (100 g)
- 1/4 cup of corn (35 g)
- 1/4 cup carrot (40 g)
- 12 cherry tomatoes
- 12 black olives

- 1 avocado
- Extra virgin olive oil

INSTRUCTIONS

- Thoroughly wash the quinoa before cooking it to remove the saponins (a bitter substance used to make soap).
- Cook the quinoa following the package instructions. Let it cool or pour cold water.
- In a bowl add the quinoa and the rest of the ingredients. Dress with extra virgin olive oil to taste.

55. *Quinoa Salad with Avocados*

INGREDIENTS

- 1 cup of quinoa
- salt to taste
- 1/4 cup of freshly squeezed lemon juice
- 1/4 cup olive oil
- 1 chopped cucumber
- 2 tomatoes cut into squares
- 1/2 cup of parsley, chopped
- 1/2 red onion cut into thin slices
- 1 avocado (avocado) in large slices
- pepper to taste

PREPARATION

- To start this idea of vegan recipes, cook the quinoa in a pot, with about a glass and a half of water, bring to a boil over a very high heat. When it reaches a boil, reduce the heat, cover the pot and simmer for 15-20 minutes or until most of the water is absorbed.

- Meanwhile, in a bowl, mix the tomatoes, cucumber, red onion, olive oil, salt, lemon juice and parsley and when the quinoa cools, add it to the bowl with the other ingredients.
- Finally, cover everything with avocado.

56.   Raw Avocado and Tomato Soup

Avocado replaces heavy cream in this rich and hearty tomato soup that is perfect for a chilly afternoon.

INGREDIENTS:

- 1 Tbsp. olive oil
- 3/4 cup onion, chopped
- 2 garlic cloves, minced
- 1 (14.5 oz.) can diced tomatoes in juice
- 2 Tbsp. tomato paste
- 1 1/2 cup low sodium tomato juice
- 3 cup low sodium chicken broth
- 2 tsp. sugar
- 1/2 tsp. pepper
- 2 ripe, fresh avocados, halved, pitted, peeled and sliced
- 1/2 tsp. dried thyme, fresh thyme, as a garnish

INSTRUCTIONS:

- Heat oil in a large pot over medium heat. Add onion, cook, stirring frequently, about 5 minutes until translucent. Add garlic, cook 1 minute.

- Stir in tomatoes and their juice, tomato paste, tomato juice, sugar, pepper and dried thyme.
- Add broth. Increase heat to medium high, bringing soup to a boil. Reduce heat and let simmer 5 minutes. Let soup cool 5 - 10 minutes.
- Cut 1-1/2 of the avocados into cubes and add to cooled tomato mixture.
- Purée the tomato and avocado mixture using an immersion blender until smooth. Reheat before serving. (Alternatively, puree soup in a food processor until smooth. Add pureed soup back to pot and reheat before serving).
- To serve, pour soup into shallow bowls. Slice remaining avocado half and place on top of soup.

57.   *Tuscan Bean Soup*

INGREDIENTS

For the soup:

- 3 tablespoons olive oil
- 2 medium carrots, thickly sliced
- 1 large onion, coarsely chopped
- 1 stalk celery, coarsely chopped
- 1 clove garlic, finely chopped
- 3 sprigs fresh oregano
- 1/4 teaspoon salt
- Black pepper, to taste
- 2 cans (15 ounces each) cannellini beans or other small white beans, drained and rinsed

- 5 cups chicken stock or vegetable stock
- 4 cups baby kale or baby spinach, stems removed if tough
- 1 tablespoon chopped fresh oregano, for garnish
- Olive oil, to serve
- Extra grated Parmesan, to serve

For the parmesan toasts:

- 1/2 baguette, thinly sliced
- Olive oil
- 1/2 cup grated Parmesan

INSTRUCTIONS:

- 1 Cook the vegetables: In a soup pot, heat the olive oil. When it is hot, add the carrots, onion, celery, garlic, fresh oregano sprigs, salt, and pepper. Cook, stirring often, for 10 minutes until the vegetables look softened and the onions are turning translucent.
- 2 Prepare the beans: On a plate, mash 1/2 cup of the beans with a fork or potato masher. Add them to the vegetables in the pot. Cook, stirring, for 2 minutes.
- 3 Simmer the soup: Add the remaining beans to the pot and stir well. Stir in the chicken stock and bring to a boil. Lower the heat, partially cover with the lid placed askew, and simmer for 20 minutes, or until the carrots are tender and the liquid is flavorful.
- 4 While the soup simmers, make the Parmesan toasts: Toast the bread until lightly golden on both sides. While the toast is sill are hot from the toaster, sprinkle with olive oil and cheese. If you have a

toaster oven, return them to the toaster for 1 minute to melt the cheese; otherwise, arrange the toasts in a skillet over medium heat, cover, and warm for about 1 minute or until the cheese has melted.

- 5 Add the greens to the soup: Add the kale or spinach to the pot and simmering for another 2 minutes, or just until the greens wilt.
- 6 Serve the soup: Ladle the soup into bowls, sprinkle with oregano and more olive oil, if you like, and serve with Parmesan toasts and extra Parmesan for sprinkling.

58.   *Creamy Zucchini Pasta*

This recipe I liked a lot for several reasons, because it is ideal if you have a celiac child and you do not want to deprive him of the pleasure of eating a dish very similar to pasta, and also because it is a great way for children to eat vegetables without protest .

INGREDIENTS:

- 1 zucchini
- 2 garlic cloves, crushed
- 2 teaspoons of olive oil
- Salt
- Black pepper
- 2 tablespoons of water
- Grated Parmesan cheese

PREPARATION:

- Cut the zucchini into long ribbons, using a mandolin or a knife. Cut the ribbon along, so that they remain fettucinis like threads.
- Heat a skillet over medium-high heat until hot. Add 1 teaspoon of oil and crushed garlic. Add the zucchini strands and stir. Add Italian seasoning, salt and black pepper to taste. Add 2 tablespoons of water and stir a couple of minutes or until the zucchini is "al dente".
- Remove to a plate with grated Parmesan cheese and serve.

DINNER RECIPES

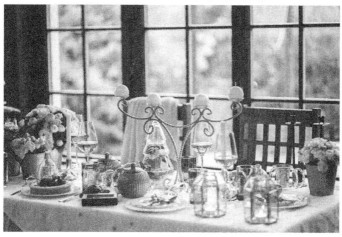

59. *Spicy Vegan Aloo Gobi*

This spicy vegan aloo gobi is super easy to throw together, has a divine flavor, and is a delicious served with rice, quinoa, or cauliflower rice.

INGREDIENTS

- 4 golden potatoes, cubed
- 1 large head cauliflower, chopped
- ⅓ cup carrots
- ¾ cup spinach
- 2 Tbsp. coconut oil
- 2 tomatoes, chopped
- ½ Tbs cumin
- 1 Tbs. minced garlic
- 1 tsp. minced ginger
- ½ Tbs. turmeric powder

- ¾ Tbs. red chili powder
- 1 Tbs. coriander powder
- ½ Tbs. garam masala
- ⅓ cup vegetable stock
- 3 Tbs. cilantro, chopped
- Sea salt, cracked pepper to taste
- Cooked brown or basmati rice, to serve

INSTRUCTIONS

- Sauté chopped potatoes, cauliflower, carrots, and spinach with 1 Tbsp of coconut oil for 10 minutes then set aside.
- In separate pan, saute ginger, garlic 1 Tbsp coconut oil until lightly browned.
- Add in all spices to pan with onion, ginger, and garlic. And cook for 30 seconds.
- Then add tomatoes and stir.
- Add in the pre-cooked potatoes, cauliflower, carrots, and spinach and mix everything together.
- Reduce the heat, add in 1 cup of vegetable stock, salt, and pepper, and cook an additional ten minutes until potatoes are tender.
- Mix in chopped cilantro.
- Serve with brown rice and enjoy!

60. Sesame Ginger Shiitake Cauliflower Rice

This cauliflower fried rice recipe with sesame, ginger, and shiitakes will blow your mind! It is easy to make, and is gluten-free, grain-free, and vegan.

INGREDIENTS

- 1/2 large or 1 small head cauliflower, broken into small florets
- 2 tbsp. sesame seeds
- 1/2 cup chopped scallions, white and green parts
- 1-inch piece of fresh ginger, peeled and roughly chopped
- 2 tbsp. coconut oil
- 3 tsp. soy sauce or tamari
- 3 tsp. rice vinegar
- 1 tsp. white miso

INSTRUCTIONS

- To make the cauliflower rice, roughly chop the cauliflower into florets, and discard the leaves and the tough middle core. Throw the cauliflower pieces into a food processor fitted with the S blade, and pulse a few seconds until the cauliflower is the consistency of rice. You should end up with about 5 to 6 cups of cauliflower "rice".
- In a wok or deep skillet, heat the oil on medium-high heat, and sauté the chile, ginger, garlic, green onions, and mushrooms with ¼ teaspoon of salt for about 5 minutes, until soft and well combined. Throw in the cauliflower rice and tamari, and saute´ for a further 5

minutes, until softened. Stir in the cilantro, lime juice, and remaining ¼ teaspoon of salt, and tweak flavors to taste.

61.   *Smoky Tomato Chickpea Soup*

This delicious tomato chickpea soup takes 15 minutes to make, and has a rich, smoky flavor and chunky texture for a quick, filling dinner.

INGREDIENTS

- 960 ml vegetable broth
- 88 g firm dry tomatoes (alone or in oil, drain excess oil)
- 20 g chopped chives (white and green parts)
- 2 medium fresh pitted dates
- 1 clove of chopped medium garlic (1 teaspoon)
- 1 teaspoon sea salt, more to taste
- ¼ teaspoon smoked paprika
- ⅛ teaspoon red pepper flakes
- 300 g fresh tomatoes in quarters
- 1 tablespoon of fresh lemon juice, to serve
- 425 g cooked chickpeas in can, washed and drained
- ½ cup of smooth parsley, finely chopped, more to serve

INSTRUCTIONS

- Pour the broth, sun-dried tomatoes, green onion, pitted dates, garlic, salt, smoked paprika, and red pepper flakes into the jar of your KitchenAid® Pro Line® Blender. Secure the lid, and set the blender to the Adapti-Blend™ Soup program. Blend until the machine turns itself off. Alternatively, blend for about 5 minutes, starting on speed 1 and gradually increasing to speed 10.
- Add the fresh tomatoes, and lemon juice, secure the lid, and process on variable speed 3 for 3 to 5 seconds until the tomatoes are just broken up.
- Add the chickpeas and parsley, and allow the soup to sit with the lid on for about 1 minute in order to warm up the beans. The soup will come out of the blender hot.
- To serve, ladle into bowls, and enjoy immediately, topped with a sprinkle of chopped parsley.

62. *Quinoa Salad With Avocado Dressing*

This easy salad recipe with avocado dressing has an incredible tangy and zesty flavor, and is an awesome vegan side dish or light meal.

INGREDIENTS

- 4 cups of black or white quinoa (cooked)
- 1 1/2 cup corn kernels yellow
- 1 cup of baked sweet potato in the oven
- 1 cup cherry tomatoes or grape tomatoes
- 1/4 cup of finely chopped cilantro

- 1 finely chopped onion cambray (substitutable by 1/4 cup of red onion)
- juice of 1 lemon
- salt to taste

Avocado dressing:

- 1/4 cup of water
- 1 clove garlic
- 1/2 ripe avocado
- 1/4 cup of Indian nuts (previously soaked for 8 hours) * optional
- 1/2 lemon juice
- 1/4 teaspoon of salt

INSTRUCTIONS

- Bake at 350 ° a cup of sweet potato in a tray covered with olive oil. Add a pinch of salt, bake until the edges are golden (20-30 minutes).
- Serve all the ingredients for the salad in a large bowl. Mix well.
- Prepare the dressing by placing all the ingredients in a blender. Blend until all the ingredients are incorporated perfectly.
- Serve the dressing on the salad and enjoy.

63.   Instant Pot Shepherd's Pie

INGREDIENTS

- 6 medium-sized potatoes, clean and broken and in quarters
- 2 butter spoons
- 680 g (1 ½ lb) ground beef
- 1 small onion, chopped
- 3 cloves of crushed garlic
- 1 can of 300 g (10 ½ oz) of chopped tomatoes
- 220 g (8 oz) of green beans (canned or frozen), chopped into large pieces
- ¼ teaspoon Worcestershire sauce
- 1 cup of grated cheese
- Salt and pepper to taste

INSTRUCTIONS

- Combine the onion, garlic, carrots, celery, mushrooms, red lentils, water, chickpeas, thyme, rosemary, soy sauce, 1 teaspoon salt, and several grinds of pepper in the Instant Pot and give it a stir.
- Arrange a 2.5-inch trivet over the vegetables and place a 7-inch oven-safe bowl on top. Add the cauliflower to the bowl. Secure the lid and move the steam release valve to Sealing. Select Manual/Pressure Cook to cook on high pressure for 5 minutes.
- When the cooking cycle is complete, let the pressure naturally release for 10 minutes, then move the steam release valve to Venting to release any remaining

pressure. When the floating valve drops, remove the lid and use oven mitts to lift the trivet and the bowl out of the pot.

- Stir the filling at the bottom of the pot. Taste and adjust the seasonings as needed. The lentils should dissolve into the sauce as you stir, thickening it. Pour the cooked cauliflower into a large bowl and use a fork or potato masher to mash it until smooth. Generously season the mash with salt and pepper.
- To serve, spoon the warm filling into bowls and top each with mashed cauliflower. Garnish with fresh herb sprigs and a final grind of pepper. Store leftovers in two separate airtight containers—for the filling and the cauliflower mash—in the fridge for 5 days.

64. Raw Broccoli Pesto with Zucchini Noodles

This raw broccoli basil pesto with zucchini noodles is vegan, gluten-free, grain-free, and is super easy and delicious. You'd never know it was dairy-free.

INGREDIENTS

For the pesto:

- 1 cup (170 grams) green peas, thawed if frozen, or use fresh
- 3 cups (100 grams) raw spinach
- 4 tbsp (60 mL) fresh lemon juice
- 1 cup (30 grams) fresh basil
- 4 tbsp (16 grams) nutritional yeast

- 4 cloves (18 grams) garlic
- 3 tbsp (45 mL) water
- 1/3 cup (30 grams) raw cashews
- 1/2 – 1 tsp sea salt, to taste

For the zoodles and broccoli:

- 4–5 medium zucchinis (1000 grams), spiral sliced into noodles
- 6 cups (600 grams) raw broccoli, chopped and then steamed

INSTRUCTIONS

- To make the pesto, add all of the ingredients to a food processed or high-powered blender and mix until smooth and creamy.
- To make the zoodles, using a spiralizer, make thick noodles out of the zucchini.
- Heat a non-stick pan over medium-high then add the zucchini noodles and cook for 2-3 minutes until tender. Do not overcook. They should still be a little crunchy but still tender to the bite
- Let them sit in the pan for a few minutes then strain them to remove any excess water.
- Add to the zoodles to a bowl, mix in the pesto and steamed broccoli and serve immediately.

65. Vegan King Oyster Mushroom "Scallops"

These vegan king oyster mushroom scallops have an incredible texture that is pretty close to conventional scallops. Just amazing!

INGREDIENTS

For The King Oyster Mushroom Scallops:

- Stems of 4 king oyster mushrooms, rinsed and cut into 1 – 1 1/2" sections (I got about 4 pieces from each stem)
- 1 c. vegetable broth
- 1/4 c. white wine
- 1 Tbsp. vegan butter
- 2 cloves of garlic, minced
- 1 shallot, minced

For The Pasta:

- 4 oz. uncooked gluten-free pasta (approx. 2 c. cooked), cook according to package
- 1 c. vegetable broth
- 1/4 c. white wine
- 1 clove garlic, minced
- 1/2 c. fresh tomatoes, cut into small cubes or 2 Tbsp. sun-dried tomatoes, drained from the oil and chopped
- 1/4 c. fresh parsley, finely chopped
- 1 Tbsp. red pepper flakes

INSTRUCTIONS

- In hot water, soak the mushroom stems for 1-2 hours. Drain completely.
- On medium-high, place the mushroom stems into a skillet. Add the broth and white wine to the skillet, getting the liquid to a simmering boil. Allow the mushroom stems to absorb the liquid completely (might take about 12-15 minutes) Please note that they will shrink in size a little once cooked.

- Toss in 1 Tbsp. vegan butter, garlic, and shallot and nicely brown the stems on each side, making sure you don't burn the garlic and shallot. Remove from heat and place the "scallops" on a plate. Keep the garlic and shallots in the pan for the pasta.
- Add the vegetable broth, wine, and minced garlic in your skillet used for the mushrooms and allow to simmer over medium heat until half of the liquid is absorbed.
- Mix in the tomatoes, parsley and pepper flakes into the skillet. Simmer for another minute and then add the cooked and drained pasta. Allow the liquid to almost completely absorb (you want the bottom of the pan to be lightly coated with liquid).
- Divide the pasta into two 1 c. servings (I know, the correct serving size is 1/2 c. but who doesn't love more pasta?!) and divide the "scallops" equally on top. Garnish with more fresh parsley.

66.   *Roasted carrot soup*

This easy roasted carrot soup is rich, creamy, and delicious, and is gluten free, dairy free, allergy-free, and paleo-friendly for a simple starter or meal.

INGREDIENTS:

- 8-10 thin carrots
- 4-6 tablespoons of olive oil
- 4 cups of chicken broth
- 1 1/2 tablespoon of grated ginger
- 2 chopped shallots
- 2 cloves of garlic, chopped
- Ground pepper
- Salt

INSTRUCTIONS

- Preheat your oven to 425°F (220°C).
- Place the carrots, onion, and garlic cloves on a large rimmed baking sheet and toss with the oil and sweetener to coat. Spread out the vegetables into a single layer.
- Roast for 20 minutes. Stir and spread the vegetables back into a single layer. Roast for 20 to 25 more minutes, or until soft and browned around the edges, but not burned.
- Transfer the roasted vegetables to your blender, add the broth, and blast on high for 30 to 60 seconds until smooth.
- Transfer the carrot mixture into a large saucepan over medium-low heat. Stir in the coconut milk and the

desired amount of water to thin. Season with salt and pepper to taste. Warm until heated through.

- To serve, ladle into bowls, and garnish with a swirl of coconut cream and a sprinkle of parsley.

67. *Artichoke Lentil Stew*

This lentil stew with artichokes is vegan, gluten free, and really delicious. This is a fantastic super easy vegetarian dish the whole family can enjoy.

INGREDIENTS

- 4 cloves of garlic
- 1 sweet onion
- 1 branch of celery
- 1 leek
- 1/2 sweet potato
- 1 not very large potato
- 2 carrots
- 1 small zucchini
- 1 ripe tomato
- 300-400g. of frozen artichoke
- 1 cup of brown rice
- 1 cup of pardina lentil
- 1/2 c. of turmeric
- 1/2 c. of spicy curry (or normal curry)
- salt and black pepper
- 3 tablespoons of aove
- 1 bay leaf

- 1 slice of lemon

INSTRUCTIONS

- To make the stew, heat the olive oil over medium heat in a large pot. Add the onion and carrot, and sauté for about 5 minutes until tender. Add the garlic, oregano, basil, and bay leaf, and sauté for about 1 minute until the garlic is fragrant. Add the broth, artichoke hearts, lentils, kale, salt, and pepper. Bring to a simmer, and gently cook for 10 minutes until the lentils are tender but still hold their shape. Add the asparagus and cook 5 minutes more. Add the peas and cook for another 3 minutes until bright green and tender. When the stew is done, remove the bay leaf; it will be thick and stew-like, not brothy. Add salt and pepper to taste.
- To make the salsa verde, mix together all of the salsa ingredients in a bowl. Add lemon zest, salt, and pepper to taste.
- To serve, ladle stew into large shallow bowls, and top with a couple of generous spoonfuls of salsa verde. Pass additional salsa at the table.

68.   *Portobello burgers (vegetarian)*

INGREDIENTS

Burgers:

- 2 hamburger buns
- 2 portobello mushrooms
- ½ tomato, sliced

- 3 sheets of lettuce, disinfected
- 80 gr strand cheese - Oaxaca
- ½ avocado, sliced
- Mayonnaise, to taste

Marinada:

- ⅓ cup olive oil
- 4 tablespoons balsamic vinegar
- 1 tablespoon garlic, finely chopped

Caramelized onions with balsamic:

- ½ large white onion, filleted
- 1 tablespoon butter without salt
- 1 tablespoon balsamic vinegar
- 1 tablespoon brown sugar or mash
- ¼ cup natural water
- Salt and pepper to taste

INSTRUCTIONS

- Preheat the oven to 450°F (232°C).
- In a bowl, mix the broth, vinegar, mustard, salt, thyme, rosemary, and garlic powder, and whisk well until combined.
- Place the portobello mushrooms in a shallow baking dish, and pour the marinade over the top. Allow the mushrooms to marinate while you prepare the zucchini.
- Cut the zucchini in half width-wise. Cut a thin slice off of each long edge so that some of the skin is gone.

Then slice each half lengthwise into 4 equal strips. You should have 8 flat rectangles.

- Make the zucchini batter by whisking the almond flour and milk in a bowl until a thick batter forms.

- Make the zucchini breading by mixing together the cornmeal, flour, bread crumbs, salt, thyme, rosemary and garlic powder in a shallow baking dish.

- Using one hand for the batter and one for breading (this helps avoid clumping of the breading), dip each zucchini piece in the batter, then place it in the breading dish and cover it with the breading. Then place each piece on a parchment-lined cookie sheet.

- When you're done, place the mushrooms on a parchment-lined cookie sheet (use the same one if there is room). Bake the zucchini and mushrooms for 15 to 20 minutes. Check at 15 minutes and remove the mushrooms if they are done. Continue to bake the zucchini pieces until they're crispy, about 5 to 7 minutes.

- While the vegetables are baking, make the rosemary thyme mayo. Mix the mayo with the thyme, rosemary and vinegar. Set it aside for serving.

- Serve using two portobello mushrooms as buns. Slather one of the mushrooms with 1 tablespoon (15 ml) of rosemary thyme mayo. Fill the buns with the crispy zucchini, sliced red onion, microgreens and avocado.

69.   *Vegan White Bean Chili*

This easy vegan white bean chili is pure comfort food.This gluten-free, vegetarian recipe is a delicious hearty meal the whole family can enjoy for dinner.

INGREDIENTS

- 300 gr. cooked beans
- 1 onion
- 2-3 carrots
- 1 handful cilantro
- 1 piece red pepper
- 1 cup fried tomato
- 2 cups vegetable broth
- 2-3 cloves of garlic
- 1 squirt lime juice
- 1 cda chili flakes
- 1-2 cdta sal see notes
- 1 tsp pepper
- 1 avocado
- 1 tbsp cocoa pure defatted see notes

INSTRUCTIONS

- Add chopped onion, garlic, cilantro, carrot and pepper to a pot with a little vegetable broth. Cook 5-10 minutes until the vegetables begin to soften.
- Add spices, broth, tomato sauce and cooked beans. Cook about 15 minutes, until the vegetables are tender.
- Pour half of the chili into your blender and beat until you have a smooth cream. Pour it back into the pot and mix.
- Add cilantro and avocado and season with salt and lime juice.

70.   *Avocado Toast with Roasted Eggplant*

INGREDIENTS

- 150 grams of avocado (heavy only the pulp)
- 100 grams of roasted eggplant (peeled)
- 35 grams of fresh onion
- 50 grams of ripe tomato
- a splash of natural lemon juice
- 3 sprigs of fresh coriander
- c / n of salt
- c / n sriracha (optional)
- c / n ground chili
- a few cubes of avocado for presentation

INSTRUCTION

- Preheat your oven to 375°F/190°C.
- Line a baking tray with parchment paper or a non-stick sheet, and place the eggplant halves cut side up

and the garlic cloves on the tray. Brush each eggplant piece with 1 tablespoon of olive oil and 1/8 teaspoon of salt.

- Roast the eggplant and garlic for about 30 minutes, until the eggplant is soft and golden.
- While the eggplant is cooking, make the dukkah. Throw the hazelnuts, cumin, coriander, thyme, salt, and cayenne into the small bowl of a food processor fitted with the s blade, and pulse a few times until the hazelnuts are roughly ground with a bit of texture. Transfer the mixture to a small bowl, and stir in the sesame seeds until well combined. Set aside.
- Once the eggplant is cooked, slice each half into bite-sized pieces, and squeeze the garlic out of the skins and mash.
- Toast the bread, and assemble the toppings.
- Mash the avocado with 1 tablespoon of the lime juice, 2 tablespoons of the dukkah, and 1/4 teaspoon of the salt.
- To assemble the toasts, smear the roasted garlic on each slice, then the avocado mixture, top with spinach, eggplant slices, chiffonaded basil, a sprinkle of dukkah and salt, and a squeeze of lime juice.

71.   *Brown Rice Bowl with Curry Sauce*

Cook this delicious recipe of brown rice with curry. It's a different option that will surprise everyone, and it's super simple!

INGREDIENTS

- 1 cup Brown rice
- 2 1/2 cups Water
- 2 teaspoons Curry yellow powder
- 1 Cambray onion , in slanted cut
- 1 cup Spinach leaves
- 1 Carrot , julienne
- 1 tablespoon Olive Oil
- 1/4 cup peanuts
- Salt and pepper to taste

INSTRUCTION

- HEAT the water in a saucepan and when it boils, add the curry. Dissolve and cook until flavored and painted.
- ADD rice. Cover and cook over medium heat until cooked. Reservation.
- MIX the rest of the ingredients in a bowl and add the rice. Salt pepper.
- SERVE and decorate with chopped peanuts.

TIPS

- The curry being a mixture of different spices, stimulates the immune system, helps improve the blood supply to the brain and speeds up the metabolism.

- Prefers brown rice for the large amounts of fiber it contains, it helps your digestive system, makes you feel satisfied and maintains the balance of glucose in the blood.
- Spinach, in addition to containing large amounts of iron, are rich in calcium and vitamin K that help to coagulate the blood properly.

72.   *Chicken Noodle Soup*

The chicken soup with noodles is a classic of all cuisines.This spoon dish retains the spirit of traditions. Chicken is a white meat easy to digest and obtain, throughout history it has become one of the most recurrent, common in most cultures and exempt from any prohibition. In the universe of the broths , it is an essential ingredient that also allows us to enjoy its boiled meat to perfection. The grandmothers say that this chicken soup with noodles cures any cold and they may be right. If you want to take care of yourself from within, take note of this wonderful chicken soup with noodles.

INGREDIENTS:

- 1 kilo of chicken
- 2 liters of water
- 100 gr of onion
- 1 carrot
- 1 leek

- 2 hard boiled eggs
- Noodle soup pasta 200 gr

INSTRUCTIONS

- Wrap the tofu in paper towel, and pat dry until all of the excess moisture has been removed. Wrap in a dry piece of paper towel, and allow to sit.
- In a saucepan, cook the pasta according to the manufacturer's instructions. Drain, and set aside.
- Unwrap the tofu, and cut the block into equal 1-inch cubes.
- In a bowl, combine 2 tablespoons of the olive oil with 1 1/2 tablespoons of the chicken-flavored powder, garlic powder, and onion powder, and stir until well combined. Toss the tofu cubes in the oil mixture until evenly coated.
- In a large skillet over medium heat, sauté the tofu cubes for about 10 minutes until lightly browned, turning when needed.
- In a large stockpot over medium heat, warm the remaining 2 tablespoons olive oil, and sauté the onions, garlic, thyme, celery, and carrots for about 5 minutes, until the onions are soft and translucent, and the celery and carrots are softened, but not browned.
- Pour in the broth and the remaining 1/2 tablespoon of the seasoning powder, and bring to a boil. Reduce the heat to medium, and simmer for about 5 minutes, until the carrot is just tender. Stir in the lemon juice, tamari, and parsley, add the cooked noodles and tofu, and season with pepper to taste.

- Serve topped with a sprinkle of additional chopped parsley.

73.   *Indian Chickpea Crepes*

These gluten-free, vegan savory Indian crepes are super easy.They're fantastic served with curries and chutneys.

INGREDIENTS

- 1 1/3 cups (150 grams) chickpea flour
- 1 cup water
- 1 green finger chili
- 1 cup fresh cilantro leaves, loosely packed
- 1 inch fresh ginger
- 2 teaspoons salt
- 1/2 teaspoon chili powder
- Oil cooking spray

INSTRUCTIONS

- In a large mixing bowl, place the besan, salt, chilli powder. Chop finely the chilli and coriander [cilantro] and toss in and grate in the ginger. Mix in the water removing any lumps that may have formed. Tactile is best – I just do this with my fingers! When you have an even smooth mixture, leave it to sit for at least half an hour or if you can for up to two hours.
- When you're ready to eat, get a tawa or frying pan to a very high heat with a drizzle of oil or a spray, then reduce the heat to medium high. Using a ladle, spoon one helping of the batter into the centre of the tawa,

swirling it round gently with the handle to get it to spread as evenly as possible in a circle.

- Cook it for 10 seconds on one side, then flip it over with a spatula and cook on the other. Remove the Pudla and start again with another one. The key is to drizzle oil on the edges of the pan before you cook the next Pudla. It can become a greasy affair, hence I prefer to use an oil spray.
- Eat hot, hot, hot dunked in coriander chutney.

74. *Potato, Cauliflower, & Green Bean Curry*

A quick and comforting green bean and cauliflower curry is just the thing for a wintertime meal!

INGREDIENTS

- 1 Tablespoon olive oil
- 1 large onion chopped
- 1 clove garlic minced
- 1 head cauliflower florets removed and chopped
- one 15 ounce can chickpeas drained and rinsed
- 15 ounces full fat coconut milk
- 4 teaspoons curry powder
- 1 teaspoon garam masala
- 2 teaspoons cumin
- 1 teaspoon salt
- 1 teaspoon garlic powder

- 1 1/2 cups frozen green beans
- cooked rice for serving

INSTRUCTIONS

- Put the olive oil and chopped onion in a large pot and cook over medium heat until soft and translucent, about 7 minutes.
- Add the garlic and cauliflower florets and stir. Add the chickpeas, spices, and coconut milk. Continue to cook over medium heat for about 8 minutes, stirring often, If it starts to get too thick, you can add a little non-dairy milk and reduce the heat to medium low.
- Add the green beans and cook until they are heated through. Season with more salt if needed.
- Serve over prepared rice.

75.   *Seaweed and Miso Salad*

INGREDIENTS

- 1/2 pack of wakame (about 1 cup dry)
- 3 spoons of mayonnaise
- 1/2 red miso spoon
- one tablespoon of sesame oil
- one teaspoon sesame seeds powder
- one tablespoon of honey
- 1/2 teaspoon grated ginger
- two teaspoons of sake
- one teaspoon whole sesame seeds

INSTRUCTIONS

- Wash the wakame with water, place it in a bowl and cover it with water for a few minutes. Follow the package instructions to prepare it.
- Meanwhile, mix the rest of the ingredients in a container until you get a homogeneous dressing. If it is too thick, add a little water.
- Mix the wakame with the dressing, sprinkle the whole sesame seeds and serve.

76.   *Soup Recipe Mushroom Cream*

This vegan cream of mushroom soup is super easy and takes less than 20 minutes! Use your high-speed blender to heat the soup or transfer to the stove.

INGREDIENTS:

- 50g of butter
- 25g of flour
- 1pote of cream of milk
- 1 liter of chicken broth
- 1 medium onion , finely chopped
- 500g fresh mushrooms , fillets or drained canned
- 1 cup of water
- Salt to taste
- white pepper to taste

INSTRUCTION

- In a large skillet over medium heat, warm the olive oil, and sauté the onions, thyme, and garlic for about 5 minutes until the onions are soft and translucent.
- Add the mushrooms, tamari, and black pepper, and sauté for 8 to 10 minutes, until the mushrooms are reduced and cooked through.
- Transfer the mushroom mixture to the jar of the KitchenAid® Pro Line® Blender, and add the broth. Secure the lid, and set the blender to the Adapti-Blend™ Soup program. Blend until the machine turns itself off. Alternatively, blend for about 5 minutes, starting on speed 1 and gradually increasing to speed 10. (To make the soup in a conventional blender, blast on high until smooth, and then transfer to a saucepan, and heat on medium-low until hot.)
- Season with salt to taste, and garnish with finely chopped parsley. Serve with crusty bread or a scoop of cooked grains.

77.   *Coconut Curry Soup*

INGREDIENTS

- 2 teaspoons olive or coconut oil
- ½ a large white onion, cut into 1-inch strips
- 2 red bell peppers, cut into 1-inch strips
- 1 large carrot, cut into 1-inch strips
- 1 cup chopped broccoli*
- 4 cloves of garlic, minced
- 2 tablespoons of loosely-packed minced fresh ginger

- 2 tablespoons yellow curry powder*
- 2 teaspoons soy sauce or tamari
- 1 ½ cups of canned coconut milk
- 4 cups of vegetable broth
- 12 ounces of rice noodles, cooked according to the package**
- 2 cups of chopped spinach or whatever leafy green you like
- 1/3 cup chopped cilantro
- 2 tablespoons lime juice
- 1 tablespoon Sriracha-style hot sauce

Toppings

cilantro, green onion, sliced peppers, lime wedges.

INSTRUCTION

- Place all of the soup ingredients into the blender jar of the KitchenAid® Pro Line® Blender. Secure the lid and set the blender to the Adapti-Blend™ Soup program. Blend until the machine turns itself off. Alternatively, blend for about 5 minutes, starting on speed 1 and gradually increasing to speed 10.
- If you don't have a high-speed blender, blend the soup until smooth and creamy, and then transfer to a saucepan, and gently warm on the stovetop over medium heat until piping hot.
- Divide the soup evenly between four soup bowls, and add equal amounts of zucchini noodles, bell pepper, cilantro, and crushed cashews. Enjoy immediately.

78. *Root Vegetable Dal*

This root vegetable dal is a delicious, hearty, protein-rich meal. Serve with grains or riced cauliflower.bread, and limes.

INGREDIENTS

- 1 cup (250 mL) red split lentils, rinsed
- 1 cup (250 mL) finely diced root vegetables of your choice, such as carrots, celery root, and beets
- 1 small yellow onion, finely diced
- 1 cup (250 mL) cherry or grape tomatoes, halved
- 4 cloves garlic, minced
- 2-inch (5 cm) piece of fresh ginger, peeled and minced
- 1 teaspoon (5 mL) ground turmeric
- pinch of dried chili flakes
- 3 1/2 cups (875 mL) filtered water
- salt and pepper, to taste
- 2 tablespoons (30 mL) virgin coconut oil
- 1/2 teaspoon (2 mL) cumin seeds
- 1/2 teaspoon (2 mL) coriander seeds
- 1/2 teaspoon (2 mL) mustard seeds
- 1/3 cup (75 mL) chopped fresh cilantro leaves, for garnish
- lemon wedges, for serving

INSTRUCTIONS

- To a medium soup pot, add the rinsed lentils, diced root vegetables, diced onion, tomatoes, garlic, ginger, turmeric, and chili flakes. Pour the water into the pot and give everything a little stir.

- Place the pot on the stove over medium heat. Bring to a boil and then simmer for about 40 minutes, whisking the dal often. Toward the end, the lentils should be completely broken down. In the last 10 minutes of cooking, whisk the dal vigorously to encourage the breaking down of the lentils. It should appear quite soupy. Season the dal generously with salt and pepper. Keep warm.
- Heat the coconut oil in a small sauté pan over medium-high heat. Add the cumin seeds, coriander seeds, and mustard seeds. Once the seeds are fragrant and popping, remove from the heat.
- Gently spoon the toasted spice oil (with the whole spices) on top of the dal. You can lightly stir it in if you like. You can also portion the dal out first and then spoon the spice oil on top if you like. Garnish the dal with the chopped cilantro. Serve the dal hot with lemon wedges.

79.   *watermelon salad*

INGREDIENTS

- 3 tablespoons of lemon juice
- 1 cup of red onion, sliced throughout
- 15 cups of watermelon in cubes
- 3 cups of cucumber in cubes
- 250 grams of feta cheese, crumbled
- 1/2 cup fresh cilantro, chopped
- Black pepper

- Sea salt

INSTRUCTION

- Pour the lemon over the purple onion. Leave to parade while preparing the salad.
- Mix watermelon, cucumbers, feta cheese and cilantro in a large bowl. Season with black pepper. Add the crumbled onion to the melon salad and stir. Add a little salt before serving.

80.   Vegetarian Ramen Recipe

This is the most incredible vegan ramen and it is gluten-free. The secret is boosting your broth with dried mushroom powder to get a real umami flavor.

INGREDIENTS

Ramen Egg

- 2 large eggs (white shell)
- ice
- 2 1/2 tablespoons soy sauce
- 2 tablespoons mirin*
- 2 teaspoons rice vinegar
- 4 tablespoons filtered water
- 1/8 teaspoon five-spice powder

Ramen

- 5 dried shiitake mushrooms
- piece of kombu (about 2″ x 4″)
- 1 1/2 tablespoons safflower or canola oil

- 1-inch piece of ginger, sliced**
- 2 cloves garlic, minced
- 5 cups vegetable broth
- 2 tablespoons soy sauce
- 2 packages instant ramen (discard the flavor packets)
- about 3 cups baby bok choy, ***
- 2 scallions, sliced
- 2 teaspoons sesame oil
- Garnish
- black sesame seeds

INSTRUCTIONS

Prepare Ramen Eggs

- Bring some water to boil in a small saucepan. Once boiled, reduce the heat to low so that the water is no longer bubbling. Take your eggs out of the refrigerator and carefully lower the eggs into the saucepan. Crank up the heat to medium-high so that the water is boiling again. Let the eggs cook for 7 minutes if you want eggs with jammy yolks. Cook the eggs for 8 to 9 minutes for firmer, but still soft, yolks.
- While the eggs are cooking, fill a bowl with ice water. You'll use this to cool the eggs so that they're easier to peel. They also stop the egg from cooking further so that you get nice, jammy egg yolks.
- Once the eggs are done cooking, transfer the eggs to the bowl with ice water. Let the eggs cool for a few minutes.
- In a small bowl, whisk the soy sauce, mirin, rice vinegar, water, and five-spice powder.

- Peel the eggs and let them marinate in the soy sauce mixture for at least 20 minutes. The eggs will soak up more flavor the longer they marinate. Make sure to roll the eggs around occasionally so that the entire surface is evenly coated with the marinade.

Prepare Ramen

- Soak the mushrooms in a bowl of water for at least 20 minutes. This will rehydrate the mushrooms.
- Brush both sides of the the piece of kombu with a slightly damp cloth. Don't rinse it under water or it will wash away some of its flavor.
- Heat the canola oil in a pot over medium-high heat. Once the oil is shimmering, add the ginger slices and garlic cook for 30 seconds. Add the hydrated mushrooms, kombu, and vegetable broth, and bring everything to boil, covered. Once boiled, reduce the heat to medium-low and let it simmer for 10 minutes. If you have more time, simmer it for an additional 5 to 10 minutes.
- Uncover the pot and add the soy sauce and instant ramen to the pot. Let the noodles cook for about 3 to 4 minutes, until they soften. Add the baby bok choy to the pot and cook them for about 2 minutes, until they turn vibrant green.
- Use tongs to remove the kombu and the mushrooms. Slice up the mushrooms to serve. I usually discard the kombu.
- Add the scallions and sesame oil to the pot and swirl to combine the ingredients.
- Serve the noodles immediately before the noodles absorb too much broth. Ladle the noodles, broth, and

baby bok choy between two bowls. Top with sliced mushrooms. Sprinkle black sesame seeds on the noodles, if desired. Slice the ramen eggs in half and add them to the ramen bowls.

81.   *Mushroom Bourguignon*

INGREDIENTS

- 2 tablespoons olive oil
- 2 tablespoons butter, softened
- 2 pounds portobello mushrooms, in 1/4-inch slices (save the stems for another use) (you can use cremini instead, as well)
- 1/2 carrot, finely diced
- 1 small yellow onion, finely diced
- 2 cloves garlic, minced
- 1 cup full-bodied red wine
- 2 cups beef or vegetable broth (beef broth is traditional but vegetable to make it vegetarian; it works with either)
- 2 tablespoons tomato paste
- 1 teaspoon fresh thyme leaves (1/2 teaspoon dried)
- 1 1/2 tablespoons all-purpose flour
- 1 cup pearl onions, peeled (thawed if frozen)
- Egg noodles, for serving
- Sour cream and chopped chives or parsley, for garnish (optional)

INSTRUCTION

- Heat the one tablespoon of the olive oil and one tablespoon of butter in a medium Dutch oven or heavy sauce pan over high heat. Sear the mushrooms until they begin to darken, but not yet release any liquid — about three or four minutes. Remove them from pan.
- Lower the flame to medium and add the second tablespoon of olive oil. Toss the carrots, onions, thyme, a few good pinches of salt and a several grinds of black pepper into the pan and cook for 10, stirring occasionally, until the onions are lightly browned. Add the garlic and cook for just one more minute.
- Add the wine to the pot, scraping any stuck bits off the bottom, then turn the heat all the way up and reduce it by half. Stir in the tomato paste and the broth. Add back the mushrooms with any juices that have collected and once the liquid has boiled, reduce the temperature so it simmers for 20 minutes, or until mushrooms are very tender. Add the pearl onions and simmer for five minutes more.
- Combine remaining butter and the flour with a fork until combined; stir it into the stew. Lower the heat and simmer for 10 more minutes. If the sauce is too thin, boil it down to reduce to the right consistency. Season to taste.
- To serve, spoon the stew over a bowl of egg noodles, dollop with sour cream (optional) and sprinkle with chives or parsley.

82.   *Arugula And Asparagus Salad*

This roasted asparagus salad with arugula is super easy, The toasted hazelnuts add crunch and lemon adds a zesty punch.

INGREDIENTS

- 100 g rocket (washed and cut)
- 100 g asparagus (cooked or steamed, al dente, cut)
- 1 tbsp olive oil
- 50 g smoked bacon (or smoked bacon, a slice, cut)
- 2 tbsp orange juice
- 2 tbsp vinegar (balsamic vinegar)
- salt (to taste)
- pepper (ground, to taste)

INSTRUCTIONS

- Polocamos rocket, heading, and asparagus, cooked and split, in a salad bowl.
- Fry the bacon in a pan, greased with the olive oil, until it is golden and crispy, reserving 3 tablespoons of the fat.
- To prepare the dressing, mix the chopped shallot, orange juice, balsamic vinegar, salt and pepper in a medium bowl. We incorporate carefully, whisking, hot bacon fat.
- Mix the green salad with a sufficient amount of seasoning, decorate with the fried bacon, and serve it tempered.

85.   *Tempeh Bacon*

This simple recipe can be assembled the night before and prepared in the morning for a weekend breakfast or brunch.Or use it for a delicious tempeh BLT with baby greens and perfect cherry tomatoes.The tempeh strips can be left marinating in the fridge 2 to 3 days. Just be sure to eat the bacon as soon as it's cooked—otherwise, it may lose its crispness

INGREDIENTS

- 1 8-oz. pkg. tempeh, sliced into 24 very thin slices
- 1/4 cup low-sodium soy sauce
- 2 Tbs. apple cider vinegar
- 1 tsp. light brown sugar
- 1/2 tsp. ground cumin
- 1/2 tsp. ancho chile powder
- 2 tsp. liquid smoke, optional
- 1 Tbs. canola oil

PREPARATION

- Lay tempeh slices in 2 13- x 9-inch baking dishes. Bring soy sauce, vinegar, brown sugar, cumin, ancho chile powder, and ½ cup water to a boil in small saucepan. Boil 1 minute, then remove from heat, and stir in liquid smoke, if using. Pour over tempeh slices. Let cool, then cover and chill 2 hours, or overnight.
- Preheat oven to 300°F. Line 2 baking sheets with parchment paper. Carefully transfer tempeh slices to prepared baking sheet, and discard marinade.

- 3. Brush slices with canola oil, and sprinkle with paprika, if desired. Bake 10 to 15 minutes, or until beginning to brown. Flip tempeh slices, brush with oil, and bake 5 to 7 minutes more, or until crisp and dark brown.

86.   *Brussels Sprouts Caesar Salad*

This caesar salad with shaved brussels sprouts is gluten-free, and is packed with nutrition and delicious flavors.The dressing is absolutely amazing.

INGREDIENTS

- 200 g of chicken breast farmyard
- 250 g of Brussels sprouts
- 2 slices of bread from the previous day
- 40 g of grated Parmesan cheese
- 6 anchovies
- 1 egg at room temperature
- 6 tablespoons of olive oil
- 1 tablespoon of lemon juice
- 1 clove garlic
- 1/2 teaspoon Dijon type mustard dessert
- Salt
- Pepper

PREPARATION

- Cut the chicken into oblong strips, season and store in the refrigerator for 15 minutes or the time it takes to prepare the rest of the ingredients.

- Wash the Brussels sprouts well. Dry them with the help of a clean cloth or kitchen paper. Cut the base and chop them in julienne with a sharp knife or a mandolin. Reserve.
- To make bread croutons, peel and chop the garlic. Toast the bread in the toaster until lightly browned. Subsequently, cut it into cubes. Heat two tablespoons of olive oil in a medium skillet and add the garlic. When it starts to smell slightly, add the bread and finish browning on all sides over medium heat, so that the garlic does not burn. Remove from pan and set aside.
- Clean the pan with paper towels, being careful not to burn. Add a tablespoon of olive oil and heat over high heat. Incorporate the chicken and cook about 2-3 minutes on each side, depending on the thickness, or until it acquires a golden tone on the outside. Remember that you can always check if it is cut in the center with a knife. Remove from pan and set aside.
- Attention: the following steps are critical for the recipe to succeed. Put the egg in a saucepan with water and bring it to a boil. Meanwhile, chop the anchovies until they are almost a paste and add them to a salad bowl next to the Brussels sprouts in julienne, 3 tablespoons of olive oil, the lemon juice, the mustard, the parmesan, salt and pepper. taste. Do not mix yet.
- When the egg takes exactly 2 minutes to boil, turn off the heat and lightly cool the egg with running water. Immediately and taking care not to burn, split the egg directly into the salad: the yolk will be liquid and the white will be semi-coagulated. Collect with a spoon

157

the remains of white that remain in the shell and pour it into the salad.

- Now mix all the ingredients with verve so that they are well integrated and the leaves are well covered by the dressing. Taste and finish adjusting salt, pepper, lemon or mustard, if necessary. At the time of serving, add the chicken and bread croutons. If left over, store in the refrigerator and consume within 24 hours.

87. *Wild Rice And Carrots*

This wild rice recipe with carrots from The Migraine-Relief Plan is a fantastic low sodium recipe that makes a fantastic vegan side dish or dinner.

INGREDIENTS

- 160 grams of wild rice
- 1 zucchini
- 2 carrots
- 1 scallion
- 1 green pepper

INSTRUCTIONS

- In a medium saucepan over high heat, combine the broth and rice. Cover and bring to a boil, then reduce the heat to low and cook for about 45 minutes. Turn off the heat, and leave the rice sitting with the lid secured for at least 10 minutes.
- In a large skillet over medium heat, warm the olive oil. Add the carrots and celery and cook, stirring

frequently, for 6 to 8 minutes, or until tender the vegetables are just tender. Stir in the cooked rice, parsley, chives, and black pepper, and stir for about 1 minute until the rice is warmed through.

88. *Kitchari – an Ayurvedic healing meal*

INGREDIENTS

- ½ cup split yellow mung beans
- ½ cup white basmati rice
- 2 tablespoons coconut oil
- 1 inch stick of kombu
- 4 cups homemade vegetable stock or water
- 2 tablespoons coconut cream

Spices:

- 1½ teaspoons cumin seeds
- 1½ teaspoons fennel seeds
- 1½ teaspoons coriander powder
- 1 tablespoon ginger root freshly minced
- ½ teaspoon turmeric powder
- ½ teaspoon fenugreek seeds
- ¼ teaspoon black mustard seeds
- Pinch of asafoetida

Vegetables:

- 2 cups of any mixed vegetables I used butternut, green beans and cauliflower

To Serve:

- Fresh lime
- Fresh coriander
- Coconut yoghurt
- Sea salt to taste

INSTRUCTIONS

- The night before (24 hours earlier), soak mung beans in ample filtered water.
- When you're ready to cook, drain the mung beans and rinse under running water. Place rice in a sieve and rinse till the water runs clear. Prepare vegetables by peeling and chopping them up, then set all of this aside.
- Heat coconut oil over medium heat, in a heavy-bottomed pot. Add cumin, fennel, fenugreek and black mustard seeds and cook for a few minutes to release aromatics, and until the mustard seeds have popped. Add the rest of the spices and stir to combine.
- Add a cup of vegetable stock, followed by mung beans, kombu, coconut cream, rice and vegetables, then add the rest of the stock (or water).
- Cover and bring to a boil, then reduce to a low heat. Simmer for about 40 minutes. Check the pot periodically as the rice swells and may stick to the bottom. Add more water if you want a soupier consistency, and simmer longer to get a thicker stew.
- Serve with fresh coriander chopped and folded through, a drizzle of fresh lime juice, spoon of coconut yoghurt and sea salt to taste.

89.   *Spaghetti Pie*

A classic Italian combination is remade into a creamy, family-pleasing casserole in this quick and easy dish.

INGREDIENTS

- 6 ounces uncooked spaghetti
- 1 pound lean ground beef (90% lean)
- 1/2 cup finely chopped onion
- 1/4 cup chopped green pepper
- 1 cup undrained canned diced tomatoes
- 1 can (6 ounces) tomato paste
- 1 teaspoon dried oregano
- 3/4 teaspoon salt
- 1/2 teaspoon garlic powder
- 1/4 teaspoon pepper
- 1/4 teaspoon sugar
- 2 large egg whites, lightly beaten
- 1 tablespoon butter, melted
- 1/4 cup grated Parmesan cheese
- 1 cup fat-free cottage cheese
- 1/2 cup shredded part-skim mozzarella cheese

DIRECTIONS

- Preheat oven to 350°. Cook spaghetti according to package directions for al dente; drain.
- In a large skillet, cook beef, onion and green pepper over medium heat 5-7 minutes or until beef is no longer pink, breaking up beef into crumbles; drain. Stir in tomatoes, tomato paste, seasonings and sugar.

161

- In a large bowl, whisk egg whites, melted butter and Parmesan cheese until blended. Add spaghetti and toss to coat. Press spaghetti mixture onto bottom and up sides of a 9-in. deep-dish pie plate coated with cooking spray, forming a crust. Spread cottage cheese onto bottom; top with beef mixture.
- Bake, uncovered, 20 minutes. Sprinkle with mozzarella cheese. Bake 5-10 minutes longer or until heated through. Let stand 5 minutes before serving.

90.   *Vegetarian ginger and carrot soup*

The vegetarian ginger and carrot soup is an exquisite preparation. It is a very popular soup recipe in those countries where it is very hot because, despite being served lukewarm, it gives a sensation of freshness to the palate.

INGREDIENTS:

- 500 gr of peeled and cut carrots
- 1/2 cup chopped onion
- 1/4 cup of orange juice
- 1/2 teaspoon fresh grated ginger
- 1 tablespoon of olive oil
- 3 cups of water
- 1 bucket of vegetable broth
- Salt

INSTRUCTIONS

- The first thing you should do is sauté the onion in the olive oil until it begins to soften. Add the carrots and let cook for 3 minutes; then add the ginger and let cook for 2 more minutes.

91.   *Cream of pumpkin and apple*

This cream of pumpkin and apple is perfect any of the cold winter days and its flavor will delight children, for its sweetness.

INGREDIENTS:

- 2 golden apples
- 1 kg and a half of pumpkin (2 small)
- 2 tablespoons of oil
- 1 onion
- 3/4 liter of vegetable broth
- chopped fresh thyme
- 1 glass of evaporated milk
- Salt to taste

How to make pumpkin and apple cream:

- clean the apples by peeling them, discouraging them and cutting them into quarters. We clean the pumpkin peeling it, removing the seeds and cutting it into pieces. Chop the onion and fry in a pan with the oil until transparent.
- Add the apples and the chopped pumpkin and sauté a few minutes. Add the vegetable stock and put the thyme and a pinch of salt. We put to boil on high heat at first and then over low heat covered for 25 minutes.
- Put the preparation in the blender and mix well until smooth and homogeneous. Add little broth if you like

thick or more if you prefer it lighter. Add the evaporated milk out of the blender and stir in the heat, without boiling.

- You can present it by serving the cream inside the pumpkin with the pumpkin seeds sprinkled on top. In that case melt butter in a pan and brown the pips. Wash the pumpkin, dry it and cut a third of the top to use as a lid. Remove the meat with the help of a melon drain.

92.   *Zucchini cream*

A very smooth soup, with different flavors, few ingredients and the final result, fantastic! The basil and curry, complement each other very well, providing color and aroma.

INGREDIENTS

- 4 medium zucchinis
- 1 tbsp butter
- 1 tbsp vegetable oil
- 2 small russet potatoes
- 1 big onion small
- 2 leaves of chopped basil
- 2 1/4 cups liquid chicken broth
- 1/2 cdta curry
- 3/4 cda salt
- 1/8 tsp pepper
- 1/4 cup milk cream

INSTRUCTIONS

- Ingredients
- The onion is peeled and cut into small squares. The potatoes and the zucchinis are washed. They are peeled and cut into small squares.
- Put a pot over medium high heat with oil and butter. Add the onion and cook until the onions are transparent. For 4 minutes
- Add the potato and the zucchini in squares. Put the fire on low.
- Cover and let cook. Stir occasionally with wooden spoon. Cook until the zucchini has released its liquid and everything is cooked, more or less for 25 minutes.
- Add chicken broth, cream, chopped basil, salt, pepper and curry. Let boil for 10 more minutes
- Mix with electric beater. Personally I like that you can feel vegetable pieces. If you prefer, you can beat more.
- Bring the mixture to the fire again until it boils. If it is very thick, add more chicken stock until the desired consistency is achieved. Rectify flavor and add more salt and pepper if desired.
- Serve in medium dishes. Garnish with lightly fried zucchini slices and basil leaf. We can also put croutons

93.   *Macaroni and cheese*

INGREDIENTS

- 300 gr of macaroni pasta
- 2 cups of grated cheddar or yellow cheese

- 3 tablespoons of butter
- 1 slice of finely chopped onion
- 1/4 cup of flour
- 2 cups of milk
- 1/2 cup of cream
- 1 teaspoon of mustard
- Salt to taste
- Pepper to taste

PROCESS

- Cook the macaroni according to the packaging instructions. Drain and reserve hot.
- Melt the butter and squeeze the onion.
- Add the flour and cook for 1 minute over low heat or until it becomes light honey.
- Pour the milk and cook for 4 more minutes or until it has the consistency of atole. Move constantly with a wooden shovel, to prevent the mixture from burning.
- Add the cream and mustard, cook for 1 minute more. Season with salt and pepper to taste.
- Add the cheese, remove from heat and stir until completely melted.
- Place the pasta in a glass refractory and bathe with the cheese sauce

94.   Onion soup. French traditional recipe

- 6 large and sweet onions
- 30 ml extra virgin olive oil (2 tablespoons)
- 60 g of butter

- 1 clove garlic
- 2 liters of meat broth
- 12 slices of baguette bread
- 3 tablespoons of wheat flour
- 1 teaspoon of sugar
- Salt and freshly ground black pepper (to taste)
- 20 ml of brandy or cognac
- 100 g of soft grated cheese (Gruyère type)

Instructions

- In a large pot over medium heat, sauté the grapeseed oil, onions, garlic, thyme, bay leaf, and 1/4 teaspoon salt, and cook the onions for about 30 minutes until the onions turn golden brown, and caramelize. Add the wine to deglaze the pan, increase the heat to high, and bring to a boil. Reduce the heat to medium, and simmer uncovered for about 5 minutes until the wine has evaporated.
- Add the Massel beef-flavored broth, tamari, balsamic vinegar, and 1/4 teaspoon pepper, increase the heat to high, and bring to a boil. Reduce the heat to medium, and simmer, uncovered, for about 15 minutes to allow the onions to melt into the broth and the flavors to mesh. Season with the remaining 1/4 pepper and salt to taste.
- Pour the Massel vegetable broth, drained cashews, nutritional yeast, lemon juice, salt, mustard, onion powder, garlic powder, pepper, and paprika into your blender, and blast on high for 30 to 60 seconds, until smooth and creamy.
- Pour the batter into a large shallow baking dish. In batches, place slices of bread into the baking dish on

one side and soak for 8 to 10 seconds until coated evenly. Turn over for another 8 to 10 seconds until coated evenly.

- Into a small skillet (that fits two slices) or on a large griddle that holds all of the slices over medium heat, pour 1 tablespoon of grapeseed oil per two slices of coated bread and fry for about 2 minutes on each side until golden brown and crispy on the edges. The amount of time and oil required will depend on your skillet and stove. Resist the urge to use less oil, or the bread won't get crispy. Transfer this first batch of bread to the oven to keep warm, and repeat the process, frying the remaining slices of bread, if doing so in batches. Keep the bread whole to serve on the side, or cut each slice into quarters or in tiny crouton-sized squares to place on top of the bowl.
- To serve, ladle the soup into bowls and top with cheeze bread, or serve family style at the table.

95. Chamomile Corn ChowderChamomile Corn Chowder Recipe

The floral honeyed tones of chamomile beautifully complement the sweetness of corn.This chowder owes its body to being half puréed, rather than to cream or butter, making it naturally vegan. I use frozen corn here, but if you're lucky enough to find fresh organic corn, by all means use it.

INGREDIENTS

- 1 tablespoon safflower, grapeseed, or other neutral oil
- 1 medium white onion, chopped (1½ cups)

- ¼ medium green bell pepper, chopped (¼cup)
- 4 small potatoes, chopped (1½ cups)
- ½ medium sweet potato, chopped (1 cup)
- 2 teaspoons kosher salt
- Freshly ground black pepper
- 3½ cups Organic Chamomile tea, brewed (about 2 tablespoons loose)
- 1 pound frozen organic corn kernels or the kernels from 2 ears of organic corn
- 2 tablespoons chopped fresh curly parsley

DIRECTIONS

- Place an 8-quart stockpot over medium-low heat for 1 minute. Swirl the oil in the pot to coat. Sauté the onion and bell pepper for 5 minutes. Add the potatoes, sweet potato, salt, pepper, and chamomile. Raise the heat to medium-high. Once boiling, about 5 minutes, cover and lower the heat to simmer. Cook until the potatoes are fork-tender, about 5 minutes. Raise the heat to high. Stir in the corn and cook for 3 to 4 minutes.
- Ladle half of the soup and solids into a blender, avoiding the sweet potato. Remove the cap from the blender lid and hold a towel over the opening. Purée until smooth. Return the puréed soup to the pot and stir to integrate. Grind in black pepper to taste. Garnish with the parsley.

96.   *Swiss Chard and Chickpea Soup*

This easy Swiss chard and chickpea soup is hearty and filling, and has incredible flavor.It freezes really well, too.This is pure vegan comfort food.

INGREDIENTS

- 6 cups drained and rinsed canned chickpeas (three 19-ounce cans)
- 3 cups canned low-sodium chicken broth or homemade stock, more if needed
- 3 tablespoons olive oil
- 1 carrot, chopped
- 1 onion, chopped
- 1 rib celery, chopped
- 4 cloves garlic, minced
- 1 teaspoon dried rosemary, or 1 tablespoon chopped fresh rosemary
- 1 bay leaf
- Pinch dried red-pepper flakes
- 1 cup canned tomatoes in thick puree, chopped
- 1/2 cup tubetti or other small macaroni
- 1 teaspoon salt
- 1/2 pound Swiss chard, tough stems removed, leaves cut into 1-inch pieces
- 1/4 teaspoon fresh-ground black pepper

How to Make It

- Puree half of the chickpeas with 1 1/2 cups of the broth in a blender or food processor. In a large pot, heat the oil over moderately low heat. Add the carrot, onion, celery, garlic, and rosemary and cook, stirring occasionally, until the vegetables start to soften, about 5 minutes.

- Stir in the remaining 1 1/2 cups broth, the pureed chickpeas, whole chickpeas, bay leaf, red-pepper flakes, tomatoes, tubetti, and salt. Bring to a boil. Reduce the heat and simmer, partially covered, for 10 minutes.

- Add the Swiss chard to the pot. Simmer until the chard is tender and the pasta is done, 5 to 10 minutes longer. Remove the bay leaf. Stir in the black pepper. If the soup thickens too much on standing, stir in more broth or water.

97. *Split Pea Soup*

This split pea soup is also gluten-free, and has fantastic flavor and is hearty and filling. This protein-rich dish is a fantastic lunch or dinner.

INGREDIENTS

- 2 cups dried yellow split peas
- 1 meaty ham bone or leftover ham
- 2 cups chicken broth
- 8 cups water
- 1 bay leaf

- 2 teaspoons parsley
- 1 large onion diced
- 3 stalks celery diced
- 2 large carrots diced
- 1/2 teaspoon black pepper
- salt to taste
- 1/2 teaspoon thyme

INSTRUCTIONS

- Rinse peas and drain well.
- In a large pot, combine peas, ham, broth, water, bay leaf and parsley. Bring to a boil, reduce heat to low and simmer covered for 1 hour.
- Add in onion, celery, carrots, pepper, and thyme. Cover and simmer 45 minutes more.
- Remove ham bone and chop meat. Return to soup and cook on low 20-30 minutes or until tender and thickened.
- Discard bay leaf and serve.

98.   *Zucchini-and-Watercress Soup*

INGREDIENTS

- 4 Tbsp. butter
- 2 cups chopped yellow onion
- 3 cups chicken stock
- 2 lbs. zucchini (about 4 med.)
- 1 bunch watercress
- salt and fresh ground pepper
- fresh lemon juice

INSTRUCTION

- In a large saucepan over medium heat, warm the oil and saute the onion and celery with 1/4 teaspoon of the salt for about 5 minutes, until translucent. Add the zucchini, 1/4 teaspoon salt, and saute for a further 3 minutes.
- Add the vegetable broth and the remaining 1/2 teaspoon salt, and stir in the almond butter until well combined. Increase the heat to high, and bring to a boil. Reduce the heat to low, and simmer for about 5 minutes, until the zucchini is tender. Add the watercress and simmer for a further 3 minutes, then turn off the heat, and allow the soup to cool slightly. Stir in the lemon juice.
- Pour the soup into your blender in batches and puree on high for 30 to 60 seconds, until smooth and creamy. (For conventional blenders, remove the small center lid cap and cover the opening with a kitchen towel so steam can escape while you blend.) Return the soup to the saucepan, season to taste, and warm it over low heat.
- To serve, ladle the soup into bowls and drizzle with olive oil. Pass lemon juice at the table

99. *Strawberry Gazpacho*

INGREDIENTS:

- 500 grams of Strawberries
- 500 grams of tomatoes
- ½ Cucumber
- ½ green pepper

- 50 grams of hard bread
- 35 milliliters of extra virgin olive oil
- ½ Garlic clove
- 1 pinch of salt to taste
- Vinegar to taste
- Water to taste

INSTRUCTION

- In batches, combine the tomatoes, cucumber, bell pepper, red onion, garlic, parsley, strawberries, and jalapeño in your blender and process on a medium speed until relatively smooth. For a more rustic consistency, pulse instead of puree.
- Add half the lemon juice, vinegar, and salt, and blend. Taste and adjust the lemon juice, vinegar, and salt to taste. If the gazpacho is too thick, add the water gradually until you reach your desired consistency.
- Chill in the fridge for about 30 minutes to allow the flavors to marry, and for the tomatoes to turn vibrant red again.
- Serve in bowls or glasses drizzled with olive oil.

100. Spinach Chickpea Burgers

These spinach chickpea burgers are absolutely delicious.Serve them on portobello buns with wilted greens for an amazing vegetarian meal.

INGREDIENTS:

- 1 onion

- 100 gr of spinach
- Thyme
- ½ green pepper
- Cumin
- Salt
- Garlic powder
- 400 gr of chickpeas
- 1 glass of breadcrumbs
- Smoked paprika

INSTRUCTION

- Heat 1 teaspoon of the oil in a medium skillet. Add the cumin seeds and spinach and cook, tossing with tongs, until the spinach is completely wilted, 2 or 3 minutes. Transfer to a heatproof plate and allow to cool until safe to handle. Drain if necessary, wrap in a towel, and squeeze out as much liquid as possible. Chop finely.

- Combine 1 1/4 cups of the chickpeas, the eggs, lemon juice, garlic and salt in a food processor. Pulse until the mixture resembles a chunky hummus.

- In a large bowl, combine the spinach with the remaining 1/4 cup beans and mash coarsely with a potato masher. Add the bean-egg mixture and stir thoroughly. Fold in the chickpea flour. The mixture should be sticky but somewhat pliable. Add more flour, 1 teaspoon at a time, if too wet, or a bit of water if too dry. Shape into 5 patties.

- In an oven-safe skillet or nonstick sauté pan, heat the remaining 2 tablespoons oil over medium-high heat. When hot, add the patties and cook until browned on each side, about 6 to 10 minutes total. Transfer the pan to the oven and bake for 12 to 15 minutes on about 350 F / 180 C, until the burgers are firm and cooked through.

SMOOTHIE RECIPES

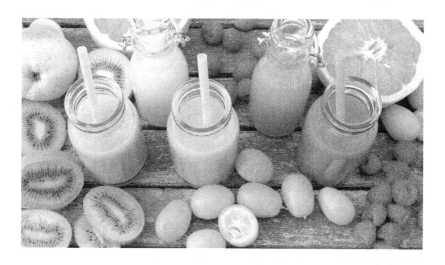

101.   Strawberry Banana Smoothie 5 Ways

This amazing strawberry banana smoothie is simple and delicious, and you can take it to the next level with these flavor variations. Try them all! They're awesome.

Base Recipe:

- 1 1/2 cups unsweetened almond milk
- 1 medium sliced banana
- 2 pitted dates (or 1 tablespoons pure maple syrup)
- 1 teaspoon natural vanilla extract
- 2 cups frozen strawberries

Variation #1: Creamy Rosewater - Base Recipe +

- 1/2 cup raw unsalted cashews, soaked
- 1 teaspoon pure rosewater, plus more to taste

Variation #2: Bell Pepper Cayenne - Base Recipe +

- 1/2 medium red bell pepper
- Pinch of cayenne pepper, plus more to taste

Variation #3: Lemon Goji Berry - Base Recipe +

- 3 tablespoons fresh lemon juice
- 2 tablespoons dried goji berries

Variation #4: Lassi - Base Recipe (Omit Almond Milk) +

- 2 cups vanilla-flavored vegan yogurt (in place of the almond milk in base recipe)
- 2 tablespoons fresh lemon juice
- 1 tablespoon apple cider vinegar
- 1/4 teaspoon finely grated lemon zest, plus more to taste

INSTRUCTIONS

Throw all of the ingredients into your blender, and blast on high for 30 to 60 seconds, until smooth and creamy.

102.   Pineapple And Beet Juice

Pineapple, carrot and red beet contain B vitamins, among which niacin.This vitamin influences the processes, such as the search for an energy source of carbohydrates, lipids, proteins and alcohol, but also in the synthesis of fatty acids and cholesterol.

INGREDIENTS

- 100 grams of pineapple
- 100 grams of carrot
- 30 grams of red beet

PREPARATION

- Wash fruit and vegetables thoroughly.
- Remove the rind of the pineapple, remove the heart and cut the pulp into pieces.
- Cut the two ends of the carrot.
- Dip the leaves of the beet in cold water to extract the juice better and cut them if necessary.
- Peel the beet and cut it into pieces.
- Insert the fine mesh filter into the SuccoVivo cold press from Imetec.
- Close the sealing nozzle.
- Start the press and introduce the ingredients, alternating them.
- Serve the juice.

103. *Orange Cream Smoothie*

This orange cream shake is a very complete drink .By combining the fruit with the dairy, makes both ingredients provide the best of each. Oranges are a source of vitamin C, vitamin A and calcium. In addition, its consumption provides fiber, potassium and a low caloric level. It is an excellent way to add fruits to the daily diet of the family and make this a success. Its versatility allows other ingredients to be added or the fruit to be modified according to taste. It is also possible to use evaporated milk or ice cream instead of yogurt and it is perfect.

INGREDIENTS:

- 1 natural skimmed yogurt or vanilla flavor (can be replaced by vanilla ice cream balls)
- 150 ml of orange juice
- 1 teaspoon of sweetener
- 1 tablespoon of vanilla extract
- 2 cookie-type maria
- 1 teaspoon orange zest

How to prepare orange cream shake:

- T riturar cookies with orange juice with the help of a blender.
- Next, add the skimmed yogurt, the orange zest, the vanilla extract and the sweetener . You can replace the yogurt with vanilla ice cream and the result is also very rich.
- Beat all the ingredients until a uniform mixture forms and is slightly creamy.
- If you want to taste it very cold , add some ice cubes.
- Serve in glasses and decorate with mint leaves or sprinkle with a teaspoon of cocoa or orange zest .
- The ideal is to consume it instantly, so that it does not lose its freshness or diminish its properties. Otherwise, take to the refrigerator until serving time.

This orange cream shake is not only tempting, but very nutritious from every point of view. Do not wait to prepare it at home! With very few ingredients and without major expenses, you will be serving an extremely natural and nutritious option to your family.

104.　*Figgy Pudding Smoothie*

This vegan fig smoothie tastes like figgy pudding and a holiday dessert in a glass. This recipe is raw, allergy-free, paleo-friendly and really delicious.

INGREDIENTS

- 1 cup fresh spinach
- 2 cups unsweetened coconut milk
- 2 cups figs
- 1 banana
- 1 teaspoon ground cinnamon
- 1 teaspoon vanilla extract

INSTRUCTIONS

- Throw everything into your blender, and blast on high for 30 to 60 seconds until smooth and creamy.

105.　*Berry Beet Smoothie*

This berry beet smoothie is sweet, delicious, and looks gorgeous. If you think you can't enjoy beets in a smoothie, this blend will change your mind!

INGREDIENTS

- 1 cup plant milk of choice or water*
- 1 frozen banana
- 1 small beet, washed, peeled, and cut into sixths**

- 1 cup fresh or frozen strawberries
- 1 cup fresh or frozen blueberries
- Optional add-in: 1 tablespoon hemp seeds

INSTRUCTIONS

- Add all ingredients to a blender, and blend for 2-3 minutes or until smooth. This one can be a bit tricky to get moving in your blender, especially if you're using all frozen fruit. If you have a "pulse mode" on your blender, I recommend using that to get it started. Then, blend consistently until smooth.

106. Mango Lassi

This vegan mango lassi with coconut, rose, cardamom, and turmeric is super tasty, tangy; loaded with immune-boosting nutrients; and is an anti-inflammatory avenger.

INGREDIENTS

- 1 1/2 cups (360ml) raw coconut water
- 1 1/2 cup (360g) plain unsweetened coconut yogurt
- 1 tablespoon coconut nectar (or pure maple syrup)
- 1 tablespoon pure rose water
- 1 tablespoon turmeric juice (or 1 teaspoon ground turmeric)
- Pinch of finely grated lemon zest
- 1 tablespoon fresh lemon juice, plus more to taste
- 1/8 teaspoon ground cardamom, plus more to taste
- 2 cups (320g) frozen mango
- Pinch of Celtic sea salt (optional, see notes)
- 1/2 teaspoon probiotic powder

INSTRUCTIONS

- Throw all of the ingredients into your blender, and blast on high for 30 to 60 seconds until smooth and creamy. Tweak the lemon juice to get your preferred level of tang (depending on the yogurt you're using) and add cardamom to taste.

107.   Cafe Mocha Smoothie

Cafe Mocha Smoothie a delicious way to start your morning. This Mocha Smoothie is made with banana, yogurt, espresso, and chocolate almond milk. Packed with 30 grams of protein per serving!

INGREDIENTS

- 3/4 cup chocolate almond milk
- 1 banana
- 1 tablespoon ground espresso powder
- 1/4 teaspoon ground cinnamon
- 4 oz. plain greek yogurt (I used siggis yogurt)
- 1 scoop vanilla protein powder
- 1 1/2 cup ice cubes

INSTRUCTIONS

- Add all the ingredients to a blender. Blend until smooth and serve!

108. Beet Berry Pomegranate Juice Smoothie

INGREDIENTS

- 1 cooked beet (I used the Vacuum Packed Steamed Love Beets)
- 1 cup pomegranate juice
- 1/2 cup blueberries
- 1/2 cup raspberries
- about 8 ice cubes (You can change this according to how icy you want the smoothie)

INSTRUCTIONS

- Add all ingredients into a blender. Blend together until smooth.

109. Banana and cinnamon smoothie with spices

The chai spice mix is traditionally used to prepare the typical South Indian tea. It is a hot and spicy drink, perfect for cold days. However, this time I bring to RecetasGratis a version of this fresh recipe: a banana shake and cinnamon with spices chai style, perfect for hot days and for breakfast. I have used masala chai to prepare a rich and energetic banana and cinnamon smoothie. I added the spices that are commonly used to make a chai shake : cardamom, anise, ginger, cinnamon and turmeric. As a result, we obtain a delicious special banana shake with a touch of spices and an exotic flavor.

INGREDIENTS:

- 4 frozen bananas
- 750 milliliters of oat milk
- ½ teaspoon cinnamon powder
- ½ teaspoon turmeric powder
- ¼ teaspoon ground cardamom
- 1 piece of fresh ginger
- ½ teaspoon ground aniseed seeds
- 1 pinch of salt

Steps to follow to make this recipe:

- Place all the ingredients in the blender jar.
- Beat the ingredients at high speed until they are well integrated.
- Pour the banana and cinnamon shake with chai-style spices into glasses and serve. As an option, I decorated it with mango flavored coconut flakes.

110.   *Rosemary Watermelon Smoothie*

INGREDIENTS

- 500 ml of water
- 2 tablespoons of brown sugar
- 3 sprigs of rosemary
- The juice of 1 lemon
- 1 watermelon without shell or seeds
- Ice cubes

INSTRUCTION

- Throw all of the ingredients into your blender (including any boosters), and blast on high for 30 to 60 seconds, until well combined.

111.   *Berry Avocado Smoothie*

This berry avocado smoothie is packed full juicy berries, creamy avocado, and the natural protein power of greek yogurt.Make it uniquely yours with your favorite smoothie mix-ins.

INGREDIENTS

- 1/2 of an avocado
- 1/4 cup blueberries
- 1 cup strawberries
- 1/2 cup 2% greek yogurt
- 1/2 cup lowfat milk
- 1 tsp raw honey, optional

INSTRUCTIONS

- Add avocado, blueberries, strawberries, yogurt, and milk to the blender.
- Blend until smooth.
- Taste, then add honey if using.
- Serve or refrigerate for up to 2 days.

112. *Berry Protein Smoothie*

This Berry Protein Smoothie is made with 6 ingredients in 5 minutes and results in a delicious & filling smoothie! It's perfect for an easy breakfast or lunch! Paleo, Vegan, gluten-free, dairy-free and no added sweeteners!

INGREDIENTS

- 1 cup Unsweetened Vanilla Almond Milk
- 1.5 TBS vanilla protein powder (Plant-Based)
- 0.5 TBS Amazing grass green superfood powder
- ½ cup frozen mixed berries or your favorite berry combination
- ½ banana frozen
- 1 cup spinach frozen

INSTRUCTIONS

- Put ingredients into your blender (I recommend using a Vitamix in the order listed & blend until smooth.
- Serve & drink immediately for best taste!
- Recipe Notes
- This is a very versatile smoothie. I'll add some yogurt for my kids & maybe a squirt of honey. Once you're familiar with the base you can let your imagination take you wherever you'd like to go!

113.   Melon Ginger Smoothie

Melons, mint, and a fresh ginger syrup are delicious complements in this fruit salad. Cutting the melons in large cubes enhances their big, juicy flavor.For this salad, I like to use a combination of four melons, choosing from cantaloupe, honeydew, Santa Claus, Persian, casaba, or seedless watermelon.

INGREDIENTS

- 1/4 cup granulated sugar
- 3-1/2-inch-long piece fresh ginger (1 inch wide), peeled and very thinly sliced
- 8 cups mixed 3/4-inch melon cubes (from 5 to 8 lb. melon)
- Leaves from 5 sprigs mint (small leaves left whole; larger leaves sliced into thin strips)

PREPARATION

- Combine the sugar with 1/4 cup water in a small saucepan. Bring to a simmer over medium heat, stirring occasionally until the sugar dissolves. Add the ginger and reduce the heat to low. Cook for 7 minutes to let the ginger infuse. Strain through a fine sieve, let cool, and refrigerate until completely chilled.
- Just before serving, mix the melon cubes in a large serving bowl and pour on just enough of the ginger syrup to lightly coat the melons, about 1/4 cup. Toss with the mint leaves.

114.   *Sweet Swiss Chard Smoothie*

The coriander seeds are optional because not everyone has them in their spice rack. But if you do, please use them! Coriander is wonderful with chard.

INGREDIENTS

- 1 large bunch of fresh Swiss chard
- 2 Tbsp olive oil
- 1 clove garlic, sliced
- Pinch of dried crushed red pepper
- 1/4 teaspoon of whole coriander seeds (optional)

INSTRUCTION

- 1 Prep the chard stalks and leaves: Rinse out the Swiss chard leaves thoroughly. Either tear or cut away the thick stalks from the leaves. Cut the stalk pieces into 1-inch pieces. Chop the leaves into inch-wide strips. Keep the stalks and leaves separate.
- 2 Sauté garlic and crushed red pepper flakes: Heat the olive oil in a sauté pan on medium high heat. Add garlic slices, crushed red pepper, and coriander seeds (if using), and cook for about 30 seconds, or until the garlic is fragrant.
- 3 Add Swiss chard stalks: Add the chopped Swiss chard stalks. Lower the heat to low, cover and cook for 3 to 4 minutes.
- 4 Add the chopped leaves: Add the chopped chard leaves, toss with the oil and garlic in the pan. Cover and cook for 3 to 4 more minutes. Turn the leaves and the stalks over in the pan

115.   *Creamy Strawberry Spirulina Shake*

INGREDIENTS

- 2 TB heavy cream
- 1/4 c. yogurt, full fat
- 8 drops vanilla stevia
- 2 packs Truvia (optional, really – tastes great without it)
- 1/2 c. green tea
- 2/3 c. almond milk, unsweetened
- 2 tsp. spirulina
- 1/2-3/4c. strawberries, organic
- 8 ice cubes

Directions:

- Blend until smooth and creamy. And yes, those fats in there are GOOD FOR YOU and they are NOT FATTENING.

116.   *Chocolate Maca Smoothie*

This maca smoothie tastes like a chocolate malt but is so much healthier

INGREDIENTS

- 2/3 cup almond milk
- 1 banana
- 1 scoop vanilla protein powder
- 1 tablespoon Maca powder

- 1/2 tablespoon cacao powder
- 5 ice cubes

INSTRUCTIONS

- Place all ingredients in a blender. Blend until smooth. Enjoy!

NOTES

- Always consult your physician before starting a new supplement. Maca shouldn't be used during pregnancy or breastfeeding.

117.   *Tastes-Like-Pumpkin-Pie Carrot*

INGREDIENTS

- pre-baked and cooled 9" pie crust
- 1 1/2 pound carrots
- 2 tablespoon butter softened
- 1/2 cup sugar
- 1/2 cup brown sugar packed
- 2 large eggs
- 1 1/2 teaspoon cinnamon
- 1/2 teaspoon nutmeg
- 1/2 teaspoon salt
- 1/4 teaspoon ginger
- 1 teaspoon vanilla
- 3/4 cup half and half
- 1 tablespoon flour

INSTRUCTIONS

- Peel and chop carrots.
- Place carrots in large pot, cover with water and bring to a boil. Reduce heat to medium and simmer until carrots are tender, about 25 - 30 minutes.
- Drain water. Return carrots to pot. Cook carrots over low heat, stirring constantly, for a few minutes, to steam off all excess water.
- Puree carrots and butter until absolutely smooth. You can do this in a food processor, blender, food mill or with a ricer.
- I use my food processor. After the carrots are smooth, mix in sugars, eggs, cinnamon, nutmeg, salt, ginger, vanilla, half & half and flour until well combined.
- Pour mixture into prebaked & cooled 9" pie crust.
- Bake at 350° for 50 - 60 minutes or pie is set and toothpick inserted in center comes out clean.
- Cool on wire rack. Refrigerate for 1-2 hours before serving. Serve with whipped cream and enjoy

118.   Chocolate   Hazelnut   Smoothie   with Bananas

A creamy chocolate hazelnut smoothie is the perfect way to indulge without the guilt. Roasted hazelnuts, cocoa, and banana make each sip satisfying!

INGREDIENTS

- 1 cup milk, (dairy, almond, cashew, soy, coconut)
- 1 cup ice cubes
- 2 tablespoons cocoa powder, unsweetened

- 1/2 cup hazelnuts, roasted unsalted
- 1/2 cup banana, 1 frozen banana
- 4 teaspoons honey, or maple syrup
- 1/4 teaspoon hazelnut extract

INSTRUCTIONS

- Add all ingredients into a blender. Blend until smooth, about 1 minute. Add more liquid or ice to thin out or thicken the smoothie if needed. Enjoy!

119. *Blueberry Pie Smoothie*

This blueberry pie smoothie is rich, decadent, and tastes like a blended piece of blueberry pie a-la-mode. This recipe is vegan, GF, and paleo-friendly.

INGREDIENTS

- 1/4 cup full-fat coconut milk
- 1/3 cup sweetened vanilla almond milk
- 1 ripe banana
- 2 tablespoons blueberry preserves
- 7-10 ice cubes
- 1/3 cup fresh, whole blueberries

INSTRUCTIONS

- Add first five ingredients to a blender, and blend for 1-2 minutes or until smooth.
- Pour into a glass and top with fresh blueberries.

120.   *Green Start Smoothie*

INGREDIENTS

- 1 serving Vanilla Essentials
- or your favorite Vanilla Vega plant-based protein powder
- 1 cup water or Silk® Original Unsweetened Almondmilk
- 1 big handful mixed baby greens, such as baby kale, chard and spinach
- 1/3 cup tart green apple, cored and diced
- 1/3 cup diced pear
- 1/3 cup sliced cucumber
- Juice of 1/2 lemon
- 6 to 8 ice cubes

INSTRUCTION

- Add all ingredients to the blender and blend until smooth.
- Adjust the consistency with a little more almond milk or ice if needed.
- Pour into a glass and serve.

121.   *Green Juice and Almond Milk*

This alkaline green almond milk is a blend of green juice and almond milk, and is loaded with nutrients for immunity.

INGREDIENTS

Almond Milk (Makes 2 1/2 Cups):

- 2 cups raw almonds, soaked for 8 to 12 hours
- 4 cups filtered water
- Pinch of Celtic sea salt

Green Juice (Makes 2 1/2 Cups):

- 2 large English cucumbers
- 2 large ribs celery
- 3 large handfuls baby spinach

INSTRUCTIONS

- To make the almond milk, soak the almonds. Place the nuts in a glass or ceramic bowl or large glass jar, and cover with filtered water, and 1 teaspoon Celtic sea salt and splash of fresh lemon juice or apple cider vinegar. Cover the container with a breathable kitchen towel, and allow to soak at room temperature for 12 hours. (For more information read here.)
- Drain, and discard the soaking liquid (do not use this to make the milk). Rinse the almonds several times to remove the anti-nutrients and enzyme inhibitors.

- Throw the rinsed almonds, water, and salt in your blender, and blast on high for 30 to 60 seconds, until the nuts are completely pulverized.
- To strain, place a nut milk bag or knee-high piece of sheer nylon hosiery over the opening of a glass bowl, jar or jug. Pour the milk into the bag, twisting the bag closed, and gently squeezing it to pass the liquid through. Set aside.
- To make the green juice, push the cucumber, celery, and spinach through your juicer, then strain with a fine mesh strainer.
- To make the green milk, mix the green juice and almond milk together.
- Store the green milk a sealed container in the fridge. The milk will keep for 2 to 3 days.

122. *Mango-Rita Green Smoothie*

This refreshing green smoothie recipe features frozen mango and pineapple and fresh orange and lime. You can't taste the spinach, but it's good for you! Recipe yields 2 smoothies.

INGREDIENTS

- 2 cups fresh spinach
- 1 cup unsweetened coconut water
- 1 orange, peeled
- 2 cups chopped mango (I used frozen mango chunks)
- 1 cup chopped pineapple (I used frozen)
- Juice of ½ lime, more to taste, plus 2 lime slices for garnish

- Tiny pinch of salt

INSTRUCTIONS

- Blend the spinach, coconut water and orange until smooth.
- Add the mango, pineapple, lime juice and salt and blend again. Taste, and add more lime juice if desired (I like mine to have some kick).
- Pour the smoothie into two glasses and garnish each with a slice of lime.

123. *Raspberry Vanilla Protein Smoothie*

Make this healthy easy fruit breakfast smoothie.Made with berry, banana, and vanilla.Without yogurt, packed with nutrition.

INGREDIENTS

- 1 cup ice cups
- 1 frozen banana medium
- 1 cup frozen raspberries
- 3/4 cup vanilla almond milk
- 2 scoops Bob's Red Mill Vanilla Protein Powder Nutritional Booster
- 1/2 teaspoon vanilla extract

INSTRUCTIONS

- In a blender combine all the ingredients in the order listed. Blend for about 1 minute.
- Pour into glass or glasses and serve.

124.   *Simple Pineapple Coconut Smoothie*

INGREDIENTS

- 1 handful of ice
- 1 cup frozen pineapple chunks
- 1/4 cup plain or vanilla yogurt
- 1/4 cup coconut milk
- 1/4 cup any milk (soy,almond,regular)
- 1/2 tablespoon unsweetened coconut
-

INSTRUCTIONS

- Place ice, pineapple, yogurt, coconut milk and regular milk in blender.
- Blend until smooth. If needed add in an additional tablespoon or two of milk. Pour into glass.Top with coconut. Serve immediately.

125.   *Minty Alkaline Kiwi Green Smoothie*

This delicious Minty Alkaline Kiwi Green Smoothie is low carb, raw, vegan, dairy free, quick and easy to make and a great energy booster.

INGREDIENTS

- 1 kiwi , sliced in half and flesh spooned out
- 1 green apple, peeled , peeled and sliced
- 1/2 English cucumber , diced (skin on)
- 1 cup spinach , tightly packed
- Small handful fresh mint , about 10 large leaves
- 2 tsp pure honey
- 1 tsp lemon zest
- juice of 1/2 lemon , medium
- 1 banana
- 1/4 cup water
- 1 tbsp raw coconut oil , optional

INSTRUCTIONS

Blitz all ingredients together in a blender for 30 - 60 seconds or until smooth and creamy. Add more honey or an extra banana for more sweetness if desired.

126. *Nifty Nectarine Smoothie*

This light refreshing nectarine smoothie is so fabulous in the hot weather.

INGREDIENTS

- 2 medium nectarines (10 ounces total), pitted and quartered, or 8 ounces frozen peaches
- 1/2 cup unsweetened almond milk
- 1 tablespoon honey
- 1/3 cup nonfat plain Greek yogurt
- 1/2 cup ice (if using fresh nectarines)

INSTRUCTIONS

- Throw all of the ingredients into your blender (including any boosters) and blast on high for 30 to 60 seconds until smooth and creamy. Tweak the ginger to taste. Salt the rim of your glass (if desired) and serve ice cold.

127. *Cherry Pie Smoothie*

This Cherry Pie Smoothie recipe is simple to make, naturally sweetened, and tastes like the pie that inspired it!

INGREDIENTS:

- 1 cup frozen cherries
- 1/2 cup plain non-fat Greek yogurt
- 1/3 cup milk (I used almond milk)
- 1/4 cup old-fashioned oats (use gluten-free oats if making this smoothie GF)

- 1/2 teaspoon vanilla extract, store-bought or homemade
- 1/4 teaspoon almond extract
- pinch of salt
- (optional) 1-2 teaspoons maple syrup or honey, to sweeten if needed

DIRECTIONS:

- Add all ingredients to a blender. Pulse until smooth, adding more milk if needed to thin out the smoothie or more ice to thicken it, if needed.

128.   *Vegan Maple Pecan Pie Smoothie*

This maple pecan pie smoothie from The Blender Girl Smoothies book tastes like pecan pie a la mode, and you can blend it up in 5 minutes!

INGREDIENTS

- 1 cup raw pecans soaked for 2 hours or more
- 2 cups filtered water
- 2 frozen bananas
- 2 Tbsp pure maple syrup
- 2 tsp natural vanilla extract
- 1/2 tsp cinnamon
- pinch Celtic sea salt

PREPARATION

- Throw all the ingredients in your blender and puree until smooth and creamy. 2. Pour into two 8 ounce glasses and be grateful you didn't have to bake.

129.   Peach Pie Smoothie

The flavor of fresh peach pie is made into a sippable smoothie for breakfast, dessert or snack.

INGREDIENTS

- 2 cups Almond Breeze Almondmilk Original
- 2 peaches peeled, pitted and sliced
- 1 banana
- 1 cup ice cubes
- 1 tablespoon honey
- 1 teaspoon almond extract

INSTRUCTIONS

- Pour the almond milk into the blender. Add the peaches, banana, ice cubes, honey and almond extract into the blender and blend until smooth. Garnish with peach slices and serve.

130.   *Brazil Nut Chocolate Milkshake*

This raw vegan Brazil Nut chocolate milkshake is loaded with selenium and totally delicious.

INGREDIENTS

- 1/2 cup Brazil Nuts
- 1 cup Cold Water
- 1 Medjool Dates
- to taste Pink Himalayan Sea Salt
- to taste Ground Cinnamon
- 1 tsp Cacao Powder

INSTRUCTIONS

- Throw everything into your blender (including any boosters) and blast on high for 30 to 60 seconds until smooth and creamy. Tweak cinnamon to taste.

CONCLUSION

The secret to eating an alkaline diet is simple: choose to eat foods rich in whole, fresh fruits and vegetables while staying away from animal products and heavily processed ingredients. Cutting out processed foods and turning towards natural options instead provides a tremendous advantage for your health, and it's sure to keep your body balanced.

If you've found this book helpful in any way, a review on Amazon is very much appreciated and if you liked it you might also like:

"The Mediterranean Diet: (2 Books in 1) Mediterranean Diet for Beginners + Mediterranean Diet Plan" by Emma Moore

"Endomorph Diet: Burn fat according to your body type" by Emma Moore

Avalaible at amazon.com

Printed in Great Britain
by Amazon